Praise for
FEEL BETTER NOW

"*Feel Better Now* is full of useful tools to help readers live with a greater sense of joy and wellbeing."
SHARON SALZBERG, author of *Real Happiness*

"Catherine Roscoe Barr has good news: our minds already contain all the resources we need to live healthier, happier lives. The bad news is we also have brains full of obstacles, bad habits, and rationalizations. *Feel Better Now* will inform and inspire you to rewrite old scripts, build new habits, and get moving."
ALEX SOOJUNG-KIM PANG, PhD, author of *Rest and Shorter*

"There is power in pleasure, and *Feel Better Now* is your road map to harnessing it. This uplifting guide reveals how simple joys can transform your wellbeing, inspiring you to live with more ease, energy, and delight."
JESSICA O'REILLY, PhD and founder of HappierCouples.com

"*Feel Better Now* is a refreshing and inspiring guide to creating a life of balance and fulfillment. What I love most is how Catherine Roscoe Barr combines science-based insights with a warm, relatable tone, making the guidance feel both practical and achievable. The book doesn't just offer advice — it also provides a clear road map for creating meaningful daily habits. The concept of a 'micro-manifesto' really resonated with me — small, intentional actions that align perfectly with your personal goals and values."

PETER VAN STOLK, former CEO of Sustainable Produce Urban Delivery (SPUD)

"'Between stimulus and response there is a space...' Catherine Roscoe Barr has offered powerful considerations about what to do in that space. Her study and experience model a beautiful approach to considering your reactions and caring for your nervous system, growing your wisdom and wellbeing. Grateful for this work!"

JUDY BROOKS, advisor, entrepreneur, community leader

**FEEL
BETTER
NOW**

A revolutionary approach to reclaim your wellbeing

CATHERINE ROSCOE BARR

Foreword by **JILLIAN HARRIS**

FEEL

The Life-Changing

BETTER

Power of Simple Pleasures

NOW

PAGE TWO

Copyright © 2025 by Catherine Roscoe Barr

All rights reserved. No part of this book may be reproduced, stored in a retrieval system or transmitted, in any form or by any means, without the prior written consent of the publisher, except in the case of brief quotations, embodied in reviews and articles.

This book is not intended as a substitute for the medical advice of physicians. The reader should regularly consult a physician in matters relating to their health and particularly with respect to any symptoms that may require diagnosis or medical attention.

Some names and identifying details have been changed to protect the privacy of individuals.

Cataloguing in publication information is available from Library and Archives Canada.
ISBN 978-1774585979 (paperback)
ISBN 978-1774585986 (ebook)

Page Two
pagetwo.com

Edited by Sarah Brohman
Copyedited by Adrineh Der-Boghossian
Cover design by Jennifer Lum
Interior design by Cameron McKague

thelifedelicious.ca

To my fabulous husband, Aaron, and my delightful daughter, Bronwyn — our family is my greatest pleasure.

To my wonderful parents, Margaret and Keith — thank you for all the lessons you've taught me, the opportunities you've given me, and the love you've shown me.

Contents

Foreword by Jillian Harris *1*
Introduction *7*

PART ONE **THE RESCUE**

1 Learning to Rewild *15*
2 Setting Yourself Free *31*

PART TWO **THE REVOLUTION**

3 The Life Delicious *47*
4 The Magic Formula *65*

PART THREE   **THE RITUALS**

     5   **Move Your Body** *83*

     6   **Nourish Your Body** *113*

     7   **Rest Your Body** *137*

     8   **Connect with Other Bodies** *157*

PART FOUR   **REVERENCE**

     9   **Zoom Out: Lovingkindness, Longevity, and Legacy** *179*

     10   **Zoom In: Your Personal Action Plan** *195*

         Conclusion *205*

         Acknowledgements *211*

         Notes *215*

Foreword

IT WILL come as a HUGE surprise to everyone who knows me well that back in 2015, I attended a book club. I had finished my stint on the fifth season of *The Bachelorette*, had led the interior design for the Cactus Club Cafe and Browns Socialhouse restaurant chains, was co-hosting the TV series *Love It or List It Vancouver*, and was in a new relationship with my now fiancé Justin Pasutto. It will be no surprise to everyone who knows me that I did not read the assigned book for said book club. But I can never say no to a good party. (Remember, this was before I had kids, when I had more free time.) So I went anyway, with high hopes it would be more of a wine-drinking club with a side of book talk and not the other way around.

What I didn't expect about that night was that I would meet someone who would one day have a big impact on my life: Catherine. What unfolded was a moving conversation between us about life, health, womanhood, entrepreneurship, and a question so many of us ask ourselves over and over: What does it mean to have it all?

I left that night feeling warm and bubbly — from a healthy combo of good conversation and just the right amount of wine. *wink*

In the following years, my life changed tremendously: our son Leo was born, then our daughter Annie; I founded The Jilly Academy, co-founded The Jilly Box, co-authored a bestselling cookbook with my cousin Tori Wesszer; and we bought a farm. But the bubbly Jilly who always seemed to have a never-ending supply of energy and positivity started to change. It felt like the more "successful" I became in my career, the less energy I had, and the more anxiety I had. While I was fit as a fiddle, I didn't *feel* healthy.

To give you an example, 2020/2021 was the best financial year of my life, and yet I was the unhappiest I've ever been. Despite the excitement of growing my personal brand and running three multimillion-dollar businesses, I knew I was not taking care of myself. I was drinking too much; I was on my phone too much; I was irritable; I was burnt-out. I finally looked in the mirror, my face swollen, my skin pale, dark circles under my eyes, and wondered, *Where are you, Jilly?*

Fast-forward to 2023, when I had the opportunity to attend Catherine's annual wellness retreat at the Oak Bay Beach Hotel with my work team (Team Jilly). I needed a change, but I just couldn't do it myself. The timing felt meant to be. Our businesses had survived the pandemic, which was a huge relief but also resulted in my feeling exhausted.

I had been trying tirelessly to "get Jilly back" for some time but with no success. I would exercise on my Peloton bike for two weeks and then lose steam. I tried this diet and that diet. I tried this strategy and that strategy. The anxiety grew, and I started to feel helpless, tired, and exhausted with everything. I was losing my creativity, my spark — and I was irritable all the time. It felt like the work I used to love and describe as my "dream job" was feeling more and more burdensome.

I was missing the old Jilly and the things she enjoyed most: savouring dinners where our whole family was present and not on our devices, moving my body regularly, laughing with my team, and having a peaceful evening with a regulated nervous system. I couldn't know for certain if this retreat would positively impact me, but I was more than willing to try.

For four wonderful days, we learned at that retreat what you will learn in this book: how to begin observing your thoughts (*How does this make me feel?*), how to rewire your brain to shed old habits and form good ones (*Neuroplasticity is so interesting! Who knew?!*), and how to be flexible when it comes to your health practices (*I didn't make my morning workout, but that's okay! I'll fit something in later today!*).

This method was the catalyst I needed to reclaim my health and move it back to the top of my priorities list. For the first time since my twenties, I knew I would stick with my good routines. I was turning the page and starting a happier, brighter chapter.

As expected, I was a ball of energy after leaving the retreat. I was so excited to implement everything Catherine had taught me. But this time, when I "slipped" and couldn't make my workout one day or wasn't feeling great on account of a fun night out, I had the ability to give myself grace. That was the key I had been missing. I had held on so tightly to this inner critical voice because I thought that I needed it to achieve my goals.

What I didn't realize was that the inner critic in me was causing me to suffer. Every question it asked (*Am I a good enough mom? wife? boss? friend?*) caused me to push myself harder and harder until I was putting everything — absolutely everything — above taking care of Jilly. By hearing the voice when I "messed up" and choosing to be kind to myself (practicing "lovingkindness," as Catherine calls it), I found a sense of freedom I'd been missing. Practicing self-forgiveness was a huge takeaway from the retreat. I am a freer, more energetic, and happier human today because of it.

I also quickly discovered I had tremendous support from the people around me once I started speaking up about my health. When I began setting firmer boundaries to make space in my schedule for self-care (another HUGE takeaway from the retreat), my community understood. Setting boundaries enabled me to be more present, allowed me time to enjoy the little moments, and — most importantly — enabled me to have a regulated nervous system, so I could feel my best. Thanks to setting boundaries, I'm not as reactive; I'm not as emotional; I have more clarity when I'm communicating; and I'm more rational. I finally feel GOOD.

I was so thrilled by the benefits I was observing in myself, and my family was observing in me, that I decided to sign up for Catherine's online coaching circle with my mom, Peggy. Not only was it a way to have continued support following the retreat, but also I trusted

Catherine and wanted my mom, who has suffered from bipolar disorder for the last thirty years, to hopefully experience similar breakthroughs. And she did, which I am so grateful for.

Meeting weekly with Catherine and that group was so wonderful. It helped me work on some areas of my healthy mindset and practice that I still needed support with. But if the retreat and coaching circle aren't accessible to you right now, don't worry — this book can be your beacon of light. Catherine did such an excellent job packing all her wisdom into these pages. I know you will be scribbling notes in your journal just as I did when leafing through these pages!

You have influence every single day. And it's important to understand and acknowledge how powerful your influence is — because your wellbeing benefits everyone around you.

If you are feeling despair at how far away you are from your healthiest version of yourself, keep reading! I felt lost too. (And if I can turn it around, anyone can!) As Catherine says, it is possible to rescue yourself. And you are capable. We get so busy in our everyday lives that sometimes we forget we have only this one precious life! You deserve to feel happy and free, and I am so optimistic that this book will help you get there.

And remember, you've got this!

xo, Jilly

JILLIAN HARRIS, Entrepreneur, founder of B Corp–certified businesses Jillian Harris Design Inc. and The Jilly Box, creator of The Jilly Academy, and bestselling cookbook author

Introduction

*"You have to come true to yourself
to have your dream come true."*
MICHAEL BECKWITH

F EELING BETTER has a beautiful ripple effect. When you liberate yourself from suffering, you liberate others around you from their suffering too. In taking feel-good steps to boost your daily health and happiness, you're not only expanding the potential for your lifespan, but also magnifying your lasting impact by inspiring those around you. Reconnecting with ourselves through small, simple pleasures is the revolution we all need right now.

It was definitely the revolution I needed.

After finishing my neuroscience degree, I worked in the fitness industry for a decade as a personal trainer and fitness instructor at a time when the spotlight was on pain and deprivation. Long gruelling workouts and bland calorie-restrictive diets were the norm, and little attention was paid to the power that mindset and mental health play in habit formation, happiness, and success.

After spending many hours talking with clients about exercise and nutrition and watching them, and myself, fail to achieve the goals we aspired to, I became burnt-out, frustrated, and depleted. I pivoted to a career as a lifestyle journalist and was drawn to the emergent fields of mindfulness, stress management, and contemplative neuroscience. These were the missing pieces that, together with exercise and nutrition, helped complete the picture for me and for my clients.

I suddenly noticed an enduring sense of happiness for the first time in as long as I could remember after struggling with depression for fifteen years. When I pieced together the steps I'd taken to feel this good, I realized that I had a multifaceted wellness curriculum I could share with others. But as I prepared to launch my coaching practice, tragedy struck — again and again. In the span of twelve months, my husband suffered major injuries in two separate bike accidents, I had a complicated miscarriage with lingering health issues, he lost his job soon after returning from medical leave, and we were kicked out of our home when the owners decided to sell. It was a lot to bear.

The strange thing was that despite the incredible hardships I was facing, I was okay — because I'd been taking good care of my psychological and physical wellbeing. Although I felt heartbroken and scared, I also felt strong and resilient, which was historically unusual for me. I experienced what I now know to be called *post-traumatic growth*, whereby a deeply distressing experience actually becomes a catalyst for positive change. I was a changed person, for the better. And I'm happy to report that my husband and I both recovered and thrived.

I had told a few friends and colleagues about my new curriculum but decided to hold off sharing it because I was in such rough shape. However, several people, who were all going through different but equally challenging experiences, asked me to get started right away. And that is how this all began. For more than a decade now, I've shared this multifaceted approach (which continues to evolve as the science unfolds) with thousands of people through my coaching practice, freelance writing, corporate workshops, keynote speeches, and wellness retreats. Now, I'm excited to share it with you.

If you've found your way to this book, I imagine you've already consumed many more on health, fitness, and psychological wellbeing. You've been collecting information on how to feel better, but maybe you haven't taken action yet. Or maybe you have taken action but keep falling off the wagon. Consistency may be eluding you. You want a sustainable solution to feel good in your body, good in your mind, and good in your spirit.

If you have no time or energy for complicated programs, if you are seeking simple and immediate solutions, and if you feel frustrated by repeated cycles of forcefully implementing change only to be derailed, this book is for you. What you are about to learn is both an instant and a sustainable solution to wellbeing. This is a straightforward, liberating, and radical approach that has already helped many people stay on track by looking at their life within a flexible framework where there is always space to add simple pleasures, needed rest, and energizing rituals.

The tools you'll have gained by the end of this book will allow you to quickly notice when you start to get off track due to travel, illness, transition, or crisis, and easily recalibrate. You will have a guiding document, your *micro-manifesto*, to keep you cruising down the road of wellbeing, pleasure, and power.

I am letting you know up front: you might find my advice boring. Within these pages, there are no fads or trends, no cleanses, no hacks, nothing hip and cool. No recipes for blue lattes or recommendations for cellulite masks. As a researcher and journalist, I am dedicated to uncovering what really works — in the present and long term. What you *will* find is science-backed, mindfulness-based, wisdom-infused advice on how to think better, move better, eat better, sleep better, and connect better. You will also read stories and case studies based on the real experiences of my clients. To protect individuals' privacy, however, names and identifying details have been changed.

What's different about the method you're about to learn is that it's focused more on teaching you how to *practice* what you probably already know intuitively, or have previously learned, rather than complicating your life with new formulas and systems to memorize. It's a return to the basics, revealing the most beautiful symbiosis between you and your natural rhythms. You can use this method to practice anything you've ever had trouble doing consistently.

In Part 1: The Rescue, you will learn why it's necessary, and possible, to extract yourself from the distressing situation you may be in. You may lack the capacity to take on another overwhelming burden, but you desperately need to attend to your own wellbeing.

In Part 2: The Revolution, you will learn a new operating system that goes against the grain and may even seem counterintuitive: do less. Pushing beyond your capacity is not serving you or the greater good. Equipped with strong boundaries and simple scripts to help you say no with confidence to what's not serving you, you can begin to decline things that deplete you, giving you more time to fill your cup.

In Part 3: The Rituals, you will learn how to rewire your relationship to movement, nourishment, rest, and connection, using simple and efficient practices to help you feel better in an instant, and beyond.

In Part 4: Reverence, you will learn how to turn the generosity, encouragement, and compassion you have for others toward yourself. You will learn how to zoom out from the present moment — however challenging or disappointing — and look back at your life, and yourself, with reverence for the preciousness of it all.

Through the simple act of reconnecting with yourself, this book is your invitation to reject relentless busyness and use that extra time to create a life that feels more simple, satisfying, and indulgent. We all want to feel better, yet so many of us don't know how to feel better, much less how to make this feeling stick. Perhaps you've been taught that the road to wellbeing requires the enormous burden of life-altering commitments, forcing you to make painful "healthy choices" and demanding hours of time you just don't have. But you are about to learn that all it takes are small shifts to things you're already doing — moving, eating, sleeping, and connecting — for you to feel more joy, ease, and personal power. I am so happy that you are here. Are you ready to make some changes?

Feel Better Now includes exercises at the end of each chapter, culminating in the creation of a personalized document: your micro-manifesto. If you want to get the most out of your investment in this book, I encourage you to get a simple notebook to write in. Keeping a journal will make your time here the most efficient and impactful — and allow you to track your progress, with a benchmark to refer back to.

Be sure to capture anything that resonates — anything you think might be important for you to learn more about and remember. As well, I will guide you through the process of strategic repetition, which is the deliberate practice of learning, thinking, writing, speaking, rereading, sharing, practicing, and reassessing. As you do this, you will facilitate powerful changes in your brain that will help you not only better remember what you're learning, but also sustain the positive changes you choose to put into action. As molecular biologist John Medina, author of *Brain Rules*, says, "Repeated exposure to information in specifically timed intervals provides the most powerful way to fix memory into the brain."

1

THE RESCUE

An act of saving from distress

CHAPTER 1

Learning to Rewild

"The way to maintain one's connection to the wild is to ask yourself what it is that you want."
CLARISSA PINKOLA ESTÉS

A RE YOU suffering? Maybe you're too burnt-out, overwhelmed, anxious, depressed, lonely, hopeless, or numb to acknowledge that there's a gap between where you are at this moment and where you truly want to be — what you dream is possible for your life. Maybe you've been too busy to even consider what you want. Or maybe you haven't connected the peripheral tension, lethargy, and dis-ease with the inner distress that comes from living out of alignment with your true self, your honest feelings, your basic needs, or your wild nature.

I see you. You're rushed, pushed, pulled. Depleted. Trying to be good. You're nurturing, managing, choreographing, and juggling. Does it feel like you're operating outside your capacity? Of course it does. It makes sense if you feel stretched too thin. This isn't how we're supposed to live. Please know that it's not your fault if you find yourself in this situation — *and* you are the one who must rescue yourself.

Many of us are struggling with a culturally prescribed lifestyle imbalance that keeps us from being true to ourselves and going after what we really want. Over your lifetime, you've accumulated a set of beliefs that might be holding you back from becoming what that little voice inside says is possible for you. This book will help you change that. I'm going to help you shed what's not serving you. I'm going to help you uncover what you really want, understand that you deserve it, create a detailed plan to get it, and develop the motivation to *live* it.

You deserve rest, nourishment, pleasure, and joy. You, wonderful human, reading these words, deserve to act in accordance with your desires. And never underestimate the impact of the way you live your life influencing others. Feeling good benefits the world around you and is an indication that things are also good within you. When you openly pursue what delights and sustains you, you inspire those around you to attend to their dreams too.

I'm here to help you attend to your dreams by creating a plan to extract yourself from the distressing situation you may feel stuck in, just as I did with my client Olivia.

THE GAP BETWEEN KNOWING AND DOING

Olivia was a successful lawyer who had three children under the age of six when we started working together.

She had an idyllic childhood in a gorgeous seaside community, where she now resides, just blocks away from her parents, in a stately home with her lawyer husband. On paper her life looked perfect: career distinction, financial success, a lovely little family. But she was not happy.

Olivia told me that her primary goal was to enjoy her life. Her definition of a good mother, good lawyer, good wife, and good daughter drove her to excel in every area. She shuttled her children to more than a dozen extracurricular activities each week, gave each of them her undivided attention every night, organized family gatherings, and planned date nights with her husband. Like many mothers, she shouldered the bulk of the mental load when it came to orchestrating their household and family life.

She applied this same dedication to learning how to feel well. When we began working together, she was concurrently doing a number of other programs and seeing a number of other practitioners, along with listening to a generous dose of self-help podcasts and audiobooks while she walked to school drop-off and pickup or did housework.

She was stuck in the gap that so many of us often find ourselves in — the gap between *knowing* and *doing*. She had amassed a ton of helpful knowledge but couldn't consistently take the most important step to rescue herself from suffering: action. If you don't take action by applying the knowledge you have, it cannot benefit you.

Olivia's self-criticism was also extreme and, unfortunately, not that different from many of the high-achieving women I've worked with over the last two decades. I also struggled with this nasty inner narrative for years. Take a moment to consider these questions for yourself:

- Are you stuck in the gap between knowing and doing?
- Do you tend to criticize yourself harshly?
- Are you driven to succeed in all of the roles you hold (professional, partner, parent) without applying that same determination to taking good care of yourself?
- Does your life look pretty good on paper (and Instagram), but you find yourself wishing you were able to enjoy it more?

If you're like many of my clients, you may have answered yes to all or most of these questions. And if you're like most people I know, everyone in your orbit is negatively affected when your wellbeing dwindles. How can you be a kind and loving partner, a patient and understanding parent, a creative and collaborative leader, or an engaged and tolerant citizen when you're depleted? You cannot.

PAIN: PROJECT IT OR PROCESS IT

The world would be a better place if we all understood our birthright to be happy, whole, and undivided because then we'd all be more satisfied, energized, and at peace. When you're miserable and disconnected, it's harder to access your humanity — your kind, compassionate, and generous nature.

Integrity, the state of being whole and undivided, "is the cure for unhappiness. Period," says sociologist and renowned life coach Martha Beck, the author of *The Way of Integrity*. "The extent to which people will defy nature to serve culture can be truly horrifying. And because our true nature is serious about restoring us to wholeness, it hauls out the one tool that reliably gets our attention: suffering," she says.

We must stop defying nature and commit to alleviating our suffering. Suffering hurts everyone. Before I elaborate, it's important to understand the distinction between pain and suffering. Pain is an inevitable part of life that spans a great spectrum ranging from the excruciating (such as a broken bone or a broken heart) to the uncomfortable (such as pushing yourself to start exercising or to have a hard conversation).

Suffering is what you make of the pain: your interpretation of it, your relationship to it, your expression of it. Sometimes hurt people hurt others. I tell my seven-year-old daughter this all the time. I want her to understand that she has the power to decide what she does with her hurt — to process it or project it.

We all have the power to transform our suffering — by acknowledging it, by seeking support, by processing it, by choosing not to pass it onto others. When we don't take responsibility for what we do with our hurt, it's like poisoning the water that we share with the community around us — it hurts everyone. Projected hurt is creating a lot of problems on our planet: from impatience and irritability to road rage and bullying, to genocide and war. It's time to address our suffering and commit to the lifelong journey of self-healing. And that begins with changing your mind.

TURN UP YOUR THERMOSTAT FOR ENJOYMENT

As I told Olivia, if you're ready to live a better life, you have to change your mind before you can truly transform your behaviour. Your mind is where your thoughts hang out, and there are a number of oppressive forces influencing your thoughts that you may need to address.

Let's start with limiting beliefs, which are thoughts that hold you back from moving forward and may be visible to your conscious mind or hidden away in your subconscious, where you're unaware of their grip on your happiness and wholeness. Limiting beliefs can put a cap on the magnitude of what you can imagine for your career success, financial abundance, love life, physical health, and mental wellbeing.

"Each of us has an inner thermostat setting that determines how much love, success, and creativity we allow ourselves to enjoy," says psychologist Gay Hendricks, author of *The Big Leap*. "When we exceed our inner thermostat setting, we will often do something to sabotage ourselves, causing us to drop back into the old, familiar zone where we feel secure. Unfortunately, our thermostat setting usually gets programmed in early childhood, before we can think for ourselves."

As adults, we must question our limiting beliefs and "upper limiting" behaviours, especially when we experience discomfort or self-destruction following a triumph in love, success, creativity, health, happiness, or peace. "Letting yourself savour natural good feelings is a direct way to transcend your Upper Limit Problem," says Hendricks. "By extending your ability to feel positive feelings, you expand your tolerance for things going well in your life."

What does this expanded tolerance for enjoyment on the other side of suffering, busyness, burnout, overwhelm, and hopelessness look like? I like to describe it as *rewilding*: being wild and free, returning to our wildness, aligning with our true nature.

REWILD TO RESTORE

Rewilding is a movement toward

- better understanding what you need and how you're suffering,
- getting comfortable occupying more space and owning your untapped power,
- saying no and enforcing your boundaries,
- cultivating a supportive social web.

Rewilding is a process of restoration that brings you back to operating within your capacity and surrounding yourself with the community that will help you achieve this slower, more delicious life. It's a return to balance: an invitation for harmony to exist between all parts of your life.

Nature isn't rushed. In the wild, life operates at a sustainable pace. Explore how it feels for you to lead with the intention to slow down, to move with greater ease, to seek serenity. Look for ways that you can feel unrushed today. How can you reduce the difficulty of the way you live your life?

Rewilding is a process of rebalancing, of living in sync with your basic needs and wildest dreams. It's a movement toward operating in integrity with your right to more rest, nourishment, pleasure, and joy. Rewilding is a process of self-discovery, self-healing, and self-actualization. I want you to truly know, love, and honour yourself. I want you to feel like nothing on paper could match the joy, vitality, and abundance that you feel inside.

When you rewild, you accept that you deserve to feel good. You slow down and savour your achievements, build your tolerance for positive feelings, weave more simplicity into your life, and find sustainable rituals to keep boosting your happiness and health, so that you have access to feeling good forever.

But rewilding also asks you to reject the oppressive beliefs you have about beauty, productivity, parenting, sex, and love, and rebuff the oppressive systems that separate you from others and your connection with planet Earth. Today we are bombarded with more information every single day than the human brain once absorbed in a lifetime. Every day the false realities of print, broadcast, and social media indoctrinate us with the insinuations that you'll be happier if you're thinner or have fuller hair, whiter sheets, or more gadgets. It's very costly to constantly compare yourself to thousands of highlight reels.

Restoring your wild nature can help you feel content in the present moment, fulfilled by your inherent enoughness. Pause right now to *feel* that you are enough just as you are. You are worthy, valued, loved.

To rewild, you acknowledge your suffering and restore balance to your life by attending to both your psychological and physiological wellbeing. Repression is oppressive. It is wild to *feel*! It's wild to howl with sorrow, growl with displeasure, or squeal with delight. "Repression — dissociating emotions from awareness and relegating them to the unconscious realm — disorganizes and confuses our physiological defenses so that in some people these defenses go awry, becoming the destroyers of health rather than its protectors," says physician and trauma and addiction expert Gabor Maté, author of *When the Body Says No*.

There are so many things we do to *not* feel: eat, drink, shop, scroll, gamble, hustle. Are you ready to live beyond these tendencies — to express, expand, and evolve? Then you must tell the truth about how you feel and what you want. Doing so begins the process of repair.

REPAIRING THE RUPTURE

Living beyond repression means that you diligently repair individual and collective wounds. You rethink what you've been taught and uncover what you've absorbed. We're all limping around with the same wound — a rupture with our true nature — but the solution is different for everyone because of the intersectional factors each of us is dealing with, such as our gender, race, wealth, health, and geography. We must disassemble the systems that separate us from our true nature and from each other. I believe that our true nature is love, and that love is the answer to repair this rupture.

It's not your fault that you've been indoctrinated by the depravity of racism and colonization, but we all need to decry this disconnection and rewrite the script so that humankind has a new story. We must recognize everyone's right to be whole, wild, and true to themselves, and learn from the wisdom of other cultures. When we rewild, we choose to see the interconnectedness of every human, plant, and animal; to operate with a sense of stewardship; to coexist with love for each other; and to respect the preciousness of all life on earth.

It's not your fault that you've been indoctrinated by the deception of patriarchy, but we all need to dismantle this system that shames us into suppressing important parts of ourselves. We must create an environment where it's safe for men to own their tenderness and nurturing and for women to own their power and ferocity. And we must create an environment where children are encouraged to embrace their wholeness and find their own unique balance of the masculine energy (structure, logic, leadership, and action) and feminine energy (creativity, compassion, intuition, and reflection) that naturally resides within us all. When we rewild, we commit to embodying all parts of ourselves and honouring that unity in others.

It's not your fault that you've been indoctrinated by the allure of consumerism, but we all need to disembark from this capitalist speeding train. Overconsumption keeps you thinking that happiness is on the other side of acquiring more stuff and perpetuates the fallacy that there's no cost to fast fashion, factory farming, or throwaway culture. The relentless gong of busyness and acquisition keeps us running on empty and denies us necessary rest and leisure. Hustle culture benefits nobody's wellbeing. You can choose to say no to this losing race; to commit to radical community care; and to foster a culture of rest in our homes, workplaces, and world. You can make better-informed choices with your buying power and realize you can access feelings of contentment in the present moment. When you rewild, you choose to prioritize people and planet over profit, you lean toward conservation and minimalism, and you focus on taking in the abundance that already exists in your life.

Is there a cost to rewilding? Yes.

Is it worth it? Absolutely.

WHAT DOES YOUR WILD NATURE NEED?

When you rewild, you necessarily leave parts of your old identity behind that you may mourn the loss of, even though your transformation is a positive one. When you stretch yourself to expand your identity and step into a truer version of yourself, you may find yourself in discomfort. But if you don't question and move through this resistance — which often manifests as fear, self-criticism, and self-sabotage — it's much harder to keep moving forward. In some instances, you may even have to let go of anyone who can't embrace your wild self.

This journey can sometimes feel lonely — but it won't be for long. When you're true to yourself, you attract people who are true to themselves, and together you can build community to sustain these changes. When you rewild, you transform FOMO (the fear of missing out) to JOMO (the joy of missing out — on unnecessary suffering).

But you are the one who must break free from the oppressive forces holding you back; it is you who must choose to take good care of yourself. No one else but you can do this. And I know you can do this! Rewilding asks you to consider what you actually want. What does your wild nature need?

Now is the time for you to become aware of the shifts that occur daily, monthly, seasonally, yearly, and within a lifetime. It's important to recognize your capacity in each moment, and keep in mind that energy ebbs and flows, that expectations can ebb and flow. It's important to appreciate the love, success, and health you already have, and the rewards that come with new milestones of wholeness, consciousness, and aliveness.

This book — this journey — is about living with as much consciousness as possible. Only when we're aware of what's holding us back can we change it. We must reclaim our wise, wild, fierce, intuitive knowing about what's best for ourselves. We must adopt the daily practice of rewilding, of incrementally aligning with this vision for our life.

This is exactly what Olivia did. She said:

> Since we began working together, mindfulness, curiosity, and intention have been essential to move from knowing to doing. Without awareness, I wasn't noticing the thoughts and behaviours that I wanted to change. Since then, I've been thinking more about what I want and have made many small and large changes, including changing jobs, registering the kids in less organized extracurricular activities, simplifying mealtimes with a meal-planning subscription, and prioritizing self-care and self-compassion by letting go of perfectionism, savouring a shower in the morning before the kids get up, keeping a gratitude journal, making a latte and drinking it while it's still hot, and connecting more with friends.

Here's a framework to help you adopt the daily practice of rewilding so that you can live with more wholeness, consciousness, and aliveness — and better align with the vision you have for your life.

In the introduction I told you that the process of strategic repetition facilitates powerful changes to your brain. To help you do this, each chapter ends with both a review of key points and an exercise to reflect on how the content specifically applies to you.

A tenet is a fundamental concept, and the tenets of feeling better are to consider what I call the 3 As:

1. Ask
2. Affirm
3. Act

The sidebar at the end of this chapter shows you how this looks. When you stop at the end of each chapter to review the key points and consider the 3 As, you are compounding the investment of your time to create the optimal environment for true change.

NOW, IN the next chapter, I'll explain why true change is not possible without learning to liberate your nervous system.

TENETS OF FEELING BETTER: REWILDING

- Begin your rescue by identifying where you're suffering.
- Become aware of bridging the gap between knowing and doing.
- Understand that what you do with your pain is a choice: project it or process it.
- Turn up your thermostat for enjoyment by addressing limiting beliefs.
- Recognize that rewilding is a process of rebalancing, of living in sync with your basic needs and wildest dreams.

Consider the 3 As

1. **Ask:** What do you want? In your journal, write down three to seven things that answer this question.
2. **Affirm** that what you want is valid and important. In your journal, write down three or more benefits of getting what you want.
3. **Act:** Practice, and reflect on, something that supports what you want. In your journal, write down the actions required to support getting what you want, then confirm that you've completed them and how that made you feel.

CHAPTER 2

Setting Yourself Free

"One of the most difficult things is not to change society — but to change yourself."
NELSON MANDELA

I HAD A loving childhood filled with middle-class luxuries like home-cooked family meals care of my generous mom and incredible summer holidays planned by my adventurous dad. My parents also made sure I had access to a wide variety of athletic and artistic extracurricular activities. But my family also moved a lot and that was hard for me, in addition to all the challenges young people often encounter while figuring out life.

By the time I was eighteen, my family unit of mom, dad, brother, and me had lived in eight different towns across Canada and the US. And, toughest of all, we moved every year that I was in high school. The lack of a throughline with close friends, extended family, and established community was extremely hard. I didn't have an adequate outlet to fully acknowledge, understand, or express my feelings. I was chronically stressed and didn't have the tools to manage my dysregulation.

For years, I was stuck in a downward spiral, not realizing I was fuelling my descent, not understanding that at any turn I could reverse my trajectory and begin an upward spiral. The lifestyle imbalance I mentioned in the last chapter was part of my problem, but my internal state needed serious zhuzhing too. I had a strong inner knowing that I had the power to overcome my depression. I just needed the right tools and strategies. I tried a ton of things, but nothing seemed to help. Until one day, I realized that I was enjoying my life, felt hope for the future, and was beginning to live with integrity toward my true self. I finally felt *well*.

As a scientist and journalist, I had to know the source of this transformation, to satisfy both my curiosity and my desire to help others thrive. So I sat down to reverse engineer how I'd finally achieved this delightful freedom. It all started with self-help guru Tony Robbins declaring that you could change your state in an instant. This was extremely appealing advice because I badly wanted to change the state I was in.

At the time, at least in my circle of scientists, Robbins was considered on the fringe. I was made fun of more than once as I toted around my copy of *Awaken the Giant Within*. But Robbins' brilliant advice led me back to the neuroscience of state change — the ability, like he originally said, to change our biochemistry and brain circuitry in an instant — and to uncover the power I had, the power you have *right now*, to make this change.

When you decide to rescue yourself, as I did, you gain the power to set yourself free from your suffering. Let's take a closer look at your nervous system so that you understand how that power works.

NEUROSCIENCE 101

Neuroscience is the study of the nervous system — the brain, spinal cord, and vast network of nerves throughout your body — which maintains internal homeostasis, or balance. In other words, it's the system that determines your state. Through observation and experimentation, you can gain an understanding of how to liberate yourself from states of suffering by learning how to influence your nervous system. Neuroscience covers a lot of ground, but for our purposes, here are a few basic concepts you need to know:

- When you are internally balanced, you are regulated.

- When you are out of equilibrium, you are dysregulated.

- Self-regulation and co-regulation describe your ability to bring about regulation within yourself, and the ability to offer and receive that balancing energy with others.

Every day we're faced with situations that bring us out of balance. Stress is a disruption in homeostasis, and a stressor is anything that causes stress. As health psychologist and author of *The Upside of Stress* Kelly McGonigal says, "Stress is what arises when something you care about is at stake." This is true not just for life and limb, but for your ideas and integrity. Some examples of stressors are the following:

- physical danger that's internal (an infection) or external (a lion chasing you)
- emotional distress, such as loneliness, fear, rage, and grief
- illness or health crisis, such as a cancer diagnosis or a car accident
- transitions, such as moving, and beginning or ending a relationship or job
- challenging friendships, relationships, or social dynamics
- novel and unknown situations, even good ones like travelling and adventure
- traumatic events
- financial worries
- becoming a parent

There's the "good stress" (also called *eustress*) of pushing yourself to meet a physical or psychological challenge, and there's the "bad stress" (also called *distress*) of exerting yourself to fight or flee in the face of a threat. Either way, this disruption to homeostasis, also called a *stress response*, then requires a return to homeostasis, which

I call the *recovery response* (often called the relaxation response or rest-and-digest response).

Our body's natural tendency is to return to a state of homeostasis — to recover — all by its amazing self, but sometimes we get stuck in a stressed-out state of dysregulation. Plus, everyone's nervous system is calibrated differently depending on their life experience, so for some of us it's harder to find our way back to regulation. The great news is that no matter what happened to you in the past, you have the power to create a better present and future *right now* by recalibrating your nervous system and choosing to get unstuck.

You can do this by addressing the collective stressors in your life — your *stress load* — and, more importantly, how you manage stress, choose recovery tools, and seek extra support to bring yourself back to balance. You can become aware of the moment you experience a stress response and choose to activate the recovery response. In their book, *Burnout*, authors Emily Nagoski and Amelia Nagoski call this process of coming back into regulation following a threat "completing the stress cycle," which involves doing things that communicate safety to your nervous system.

You will learn many tools to do this in the pages of this book. Let's zoom in and see what completing the stress cycle looks like in your body. Stay with me as I give you a crash course on your nervous system.

MEET YOUR INCREDIBLE NERVOUS SYSTEM

Your nervous system has two main parts to its vast network of nerve cells. Your *central nervous system* encompasses the brain and spinal cord, and your *peripheral nervous system* encompasses the rest of the nerves that innervate every organ, muscle, and tissue throughout your body.

Your peripheral nervous system has two branches:

- The *somatic nervous system* is primarily responsible for conscious processes like voluntary body movements, and sending sensory signals from your skin, joints, and muscles to your brain.

- The *autonomic nervous system* is primarily responsible for unconscious (involuntary) processes including respiration, cardiovascular function, metabolism, and digestion.

There are also two branches of the autonomic nervous system:

- The *sympathetic nervous system*, which acts like your accelerator, is the system of *action*. It sends your body the signal to expend energy, helping you to fight or flee, as well as engage and achieve.

- The *parasympathetic nervous system*, which acts like your brake, is the system of *rest and repair*. It sends your body the signal to conserve energy, helping you to rest and digest, as well as causing you to freeze (when it hits the brake too hard) in response to overwhelming stress.

But there's one nerve in the parasympathetic nervous system that's captured the media's attention and rightly so.

THE MIGHTY VAGUS NERVE

The vagus nerve is the primary pathway of the parasympathetic nervous system. It's actually a pair of nerves originating in the brainstem. Named for the Latin word for "wandering," the vagus nerve does just that! From head to tail, it innervates your face, throat, heart, lungs, gut, and sex organs.

Polyvagal theory suggests the split of the vagus nerve into two branches (I know, so many branches!):

- The *ventral vagal system* supports social engagement.
- The *dorsal vagal system* supports immobilizing behaviours (whereas the sympathetic nervous system supports mobilizing behaviours).

In *Anchored*, licensed clinical social worker Deb Dana describes the hierarchical order that these three neural circuits — the sympathetic nervous system, ventral vagal system, and dorsal vagal system — are activated in:

1. connection
2. mobilization
3. immobilization

As we are social animals, our first instinct is to connect and seek or provide support. If none of those actions provide a solution, our next reaction is to fight or flee. Our last resort is to freeze.

These states work together and, says Dana, when in healthy balance can anchor us in a sense of safety with mobilizing energy (striving to meet a challenge) or immobilizing energy (curling up to rest). It's only when we lose our sense of safety (physically or psychologically) that we become dysregulated. This awareness of our nervous system can help us be more specific in identifying and resolving dysregulation. For example, anxiety is the antsy energy of sympathetic activation, whereas depression is the detached energy of parasympathetic (dorsal vagal) activation.

A healthy balance between these three neural circuits is indicated by your *vagal tone*: the ability of your parasympathetic nervous system to apply the brake to return you from a sympathetic state of fight or flee or release the brake enough to return you from a dorsal vagal state of freeze. Vagal tone can be calculated by measuring your *heart rate variability* (HRV), which is the difference in timing between successive heartbeats, and indicates your nervous system's ability to be light on its feet and quick to respond to internal or external threats and challenges.

A high HRV, and therefore a high vagal tone, has been linked to better executive function (cognitive skills like focus, flexibility, self-control, and working memory) and emotional regulation. A low HRV has been linked to cardiovascular disease, cognitive decline, and negative moods. So how do you increase your HRV and vagal tone? Put another way, how can you improve the effectiveness of your parasympathetic nervous system at reinstating a regulated state of safety and connection following a threat? Bear in mind that threats can be either physical (being chased by a bear or fighting a virus) or psychological (being overwhelmed by your inbox or having a sense of loneliness), and every one of us experiences them, in some shape or form, multiple times every day.

YOU CAN increase your vagal tone and improve the effectiveness of your parasympathetic nervous system by practicing a personal selection of the many different somatic (body) and cognitive (mind) tools you will learn about as you read this book.

Top-down tools are cognitive: you're using your mind to influence how you feel, as we began to do in the last chapter. Bottom-up tools are somatic: you're using your body to influence how you feel, as we're learning in this and upcoming chapters.

INCREASING VAGAL TONE WITH SOMATIC PRACTICES

Our autonomic nervous system communicates via two main types of nerves:

- Sensory nerves, also called *afferent* nerves, carry information from body to brain.
- Motor nerves, also called *efferent* nerves, carry information from brain to body.

Mixed nerves are composed of both sensory and motor nerves, and the vagus nerve is one such mixed nerve. The bidirectional communication of the vagus nerve is 80 per cent afferent (from body to brain). This means that you have myriad ways to send feel-good, I'm-safe, don't-stress messages to your brain and shift the state you're in. You can do this through the conscious engagement of the many body systems this wondrous nerve innervates. Here's a short list of body-based tools that can activate your parasympathetic nervous system — and help you complete the stress cycle. I'll dig into some of these more deeply in the coming chapters:

- eye gazing with a kind someone, genuine smiling, and laughing
- singing, humming, or chanting
- positive social connections
- physical affection
- hot and cold exposure (saunas, cold plunges)
- breathwork (deliberate breathing)
- physical activity (walking, yoga, swimming, running, tai chi, hiking, gardening, cycling, weightlifting)
- expressing distress (crying, journaling, unloading your woes with a friend or therapist, unloading your woes on a punching bag)
- nourishment (slowing down to savour the consumption of healthy nutrition)

- orgasm

- creative expression

Activating your parasympathetic nervous system not only can help you feel better psychologically, but also benefits you physically. Parasympathetic activation restores you after the depletion of sympathetic activation. With sympathetic activation, you gain the energy to instantly mobilize in the face of a threat. Your body does this by redirecting energy (in the form of blood sugar) from the systems that aren't essential during a life-or-death situation, such as your immune, digestive, and reproductive systems.

Over time, with chronic stress, these extremely important systems become depleted, leading to immune, digestive, and reproductive disorders. Plus, without enough physical activity to burn the excess fuel (if it wasn't used to fight or flee but rather to sit and stew), your body will stockpile this excess fuel in the form of a muffin top or spare tire. This happens to be the most dangerous kind of body fat (called visceral fat) because it surrounds your abdominal organs, releases inflammatory proteins, and increases your risk of diabetes and heart disease. This is one reason that waist size can be a good measure of overall health.

Now you can see why not managing chronic stress (either pressing the accelerator or brake too hard) is, at best, a double whammy. It's extremely important for your health and longevity to choose somatic and cognitive tools that bring you back into regulation, every day.

When you complete the stress cycle and activate your parasympathetic nervous system, your immune, digestive, and reproductive systems are flooded with the energy they need for you to thrive.

The next time you feel powerless to change your current situation, or hopeless that things will never change for the better, remind yourself of the incredible power you have *right now* to liberate yourself from suffering. The opposite of suffering is pleasure: a feeling of happy satisfaction and enjoyment. So, in the next chapter, I will show you how to build healthy habits and break bad habits by focusing on things that make you feel good and embracing life's small, simple pleasures!

TENETS OF FEELING BETTER: LIBERATION

- You have the power to liberate yourself from suffering.
- Self-regulation and co-regulation describe your ability to bring about regulation within yourself, and the ability to offer and receive that balancing energy with others.
- Dysregulation describes a state of internal imbalance.
- You always have access to tools that can help you complete the stress cycle and communicate safety to your nervous system.
- The vagus nerve innervates many of the major organs in your body, and through the use of both somatic (body) and cognitive (mind) tools, you can activate your parasympathetic nervous system and return to a state of safety and connection.

Consider the 3 As

1. **Ask:** What do you need to feel safe and connected? In your journal, write down three to seven things that answer this question.
2. **Affirm** that what you need is valid and important. In your journal, write down three or more benefits of feeling safe and connected.
3. **Act:** Practice, and reflect on, something to promote safety and connection. In your journal, write down the actions required to promote safety and connection, then confirm that you've completed them and how that made you feel.

THE REVOLUTION

2

A system overthrow in favour of a new way

CHAPTER 3

The Life Delicious

"We are all being asked to show up, find our voice, take action, honour life, participate in growth, and BE the... change."
SEANE CORN

ONE DAY, as I began the journey of crawling out of my miserable hole, I was practicing yoga, alone on my sunny patio. Because I had been journaling with parameters — by gathering data on what made me feel good (and bad) — the combination of conscious breathing, mindful movement, and brilliant sunshine really struck me as *delicious*. In what I can describe only as an instant download, the name for my new business, based on an integrated system that encompassed mental, physical, and spiritual wellbeing, and focused on indulgence and pleasure, came to me: The Life Delicious.

In that blissful moment on the patio, I understood that I had been too focused on negative experiences, real or perceived, and that I hadn't given adequate attention to positive experiences, small or large. The practice of gathering data on what made me feel good had shifted my attention and upgraded my brain to become better at doing so unconsciously. "What you pay attention to is the primary shaper of your brain," says neuropsychologist Rick Hanson, the author of *Hardwiring Happiness*. "Mental states become neural traits."

That gloomy outlook I'd been wearing is, in fact, pretty normal. Our brains have a built-in safety mechanism to protect us from danger, and it's called the *negativity bias*. The early humans who survived long enough to reproduce so that we could be here today were likely the ones who were the most highly attuned to threats.

As I discussed in chapter 2, nowadays most threats come in the form of notifications, multitasking, consumerism, and loneliness — not lions and tigers and bears — and our focus on these modern challenges can make life feel quite glum.

But we can overcome this tendency and strike a healthy balance between being vigilant and being exuberant by consciously savouring good experiences. Consciously savouring good experiences is how we rewire our brain for the better, so that we can begin to unconsciously move toward more and more good experiences — toward a more delicious life.

THE BARRIER TO A DELICIOUS LIFE

We all have knowledge and important reasons to *apply* that knowledge, but we're not doing it. Why aren't we doing it? Answering this question has been the greatest motivating force in my personal and professional life. How can the vast majority of us *know* that we need to think better, move better, eat better, sleep better, and connect better but not *do* the things that could help us live better and feel better?

I believe *the* biggest barrier to health, happiness, and vitality, and the singular cause of all of the suffering I've seen in my clients — and myself — is *unmindfulness*. Unmindfulness is the state of being unconscious, or unaware, of how your thoughts, words, and actions make you feel. None of us wakes up in the morning intending to feel like garbage. No one *wants* to suffer. But it's easy to stay stuck in destructive patterns when we don't realize that they're the cause of our suffering.

When you're unmindful, you may

- be caught up in negative rumination about yourself and life,
- tend to live a sedentary lifestyle,
- choose substandard food because you don't have time or are too tired to consider better options,
- have compromised sleep hygiene,
- not prioritize your most important relationships.

If one word describes the bulk of our suffering, then one word describes our freedom: *mindfulness*. Mindfulness is the state of being conscious, or aware, of how your thoughts, words, and actions make you feel. And when you become more mindful, you tend to make better choices overall.

On learning the practice of mindfulness, my client Fleur, a marketing director at a medical tech firm, said, "It suddenly feels like I'm in control, I'm conscious, I'm present — I'm not living on autopilot. Becoming more mindful has been one of my biggest revelations. I didn't realize how far along I was in being unconscious, or not present, until going through this program. Wow. Now I feel equipped to be more present, more mindful, and more connected in my life."

When you are fully aware of how your thoughts, words, and actions make you feel, you can bridge the gap between knowing and doing and begin *living* the life you dream of.

But how do you rewire your brain for that change?

REWIRING YOUR BRAIN

When I turned thirty, I hit rock bottom. I had been walking around in an unmindful daze for years, and I hated it. I knew I shouldn't feel miserable most of the time, but I didn't know how to crawl out of the hole I was in. At the end of that year, I was so overwhelmed by sadness that I considered taking my own life. But something inside of me screamed that I *could* find a way out, and the idea to embark on this revolution as a science experiment came into vision.

Previously, I had journaled only when I was really upset, which fueled my negative rumination, further activated my stress response, and kept me focused on my struggles instead of solutions. So I decided to write down how all of my thoughts, words, and actions made me feel in the ensuing minutes and hours. And something unexpected happened. I started to radically change my behaviour — my thoughts, words, and actions. With very little effort. I had forcefully, effortfully tried to change my behaviour for years and continually failed to do so. What the heck was going on?

The answer to that question was *neuroplasticity*, which I learned about from Rick Hanson. Neuroplasticity is the capacity of our brain to change, to rewire its connections — a capacity it maintains throughout our entire life. "Whatever we repeatedly sense and feel and want and think is slowly but surely sculpting neural structure," says Hanson.

Every day, your brain is either reinforcing or rebuffing your behaviour — whether it's constructive (helpful) or destructive (harmful) — and you have the power to take the wheel and steer things in a positive direction. "Neurons that fire together wire together" goes the famous saying from the "father of neuropsychology," Donald Hebb. Neuroplasticity is the act of forming or fracturing, wiring or unwiring, these neural pathways.

Think of a habit like a freeway: a long, flat, wide road that you can speed along on autopilot. When you try to form a new habit, it feels like bushwhacking through a dense forest — it's bumpy and narrow, and requires your full attention to navigate. But the more you choose to travel this path, the easier it gets. It becomes a passable walkway, then a gravel road, then, eventually, a newly paved freeway (where you can relax a little and crank the good tunes). And the old freeway (the old habit) slowly begins to deteriorate, becoming overgrown and impassable.

There are two types of neuroplasticity:

1 **Experience-dependent neuroplasticity** is a *passive* process that happens unconsciously, without your awareness. When you are stuck in destructive patterns, you are unconsciously reinforcing them through repetition. This is why we're able to develop strong habits that don't serve us and why we have trouble trying to disconnect from them.

2 **Self-directed neuroplasticity** is an *active* process that happens consciously, with your awareness. This is the secret to developing solid and enduring habits that serve us! Consciously harnessing the power of my brain's plasticity is how I radically changed my life — and how you can do the same.

By using my journal to write down how my thoughts, words, and actions made me feel, I was sparking the process of self-directed neuroplasticity. I wrote down how eating junk food, skipping workouts, and staying up late made me feel (terrible), and this began to unwire my brain *from* these behaviours. I wrote down how eating nutritious food, working out, and going to bed early made me feel (wonderful), and this began to wire my brain *to* these behaviours. I was galvanizing myself toward constructive habits and repelling myself from destructive habits. It was incredible.

I experienced a thrilling power that I'd never had before:

- the strength to resist unhealthy habits
- the motivation to practice healthy habits

Are you ready to rewire your relationship to wellbeing and hardwire healthy habits? One way to do this is to adopt a flexible framework so that you don't get derailed by trying to do everything all at once.

THE FLEXIBLE FRAMEWORK

Pamela, the HR manager for a large brand, was a committed long-distance runner. But she struggled to feel as good as she could while on vacation with her family because she completely missed out on the workouts that energized and elated her. She faced one of the barriers that many of us struggle with when trying to stay consistent with prioritizing our own wellbeing.

Quinn, a journalist and singer-songwriter, struggled with this barrier too. "It held me back for at least twenty years," she told me. "I have all this knowledge I've accumulated throughout my life, and I know what I need to do and why I need to do it, but I'm not doing it. I'm just stuck."

I call this approach an *all-or-nothing mentality*, but it's also known as perfection paralysis and black-or-white thinking. The all-or-nothing mentality keeps you stuck, unable to act, and stagnant, and if you do get started, it makes sure you fall off the wagon soon after. To break through this barrier, you must banish the all-or-nothing mentality, embrace imperfection, and adopt grey-zone thinking. I call this easy-breezy way of living the *flexible framework*.

"The flexible framework gave me permission to be imperfect and consistent," said my long-time client Rachel, a business development advisor. She shared with me that instead of skipping her daily walk, shrinking it to just five minutes on a hectic workday had a significant impact on her wellbeing. "If you can keep a routine, it makes all the difference in the world. That was a big takeaway that's evolved over the last ten years. The all-or-nothing mentality was a tendency to overthink and over-optimize, which could make even a healthy choice feel heavy instead of light."

So what does the flexible framework look like? Here are three points of departure from the all-or-nothing mentality you can adopt:

1 **Your habits can expand or contract:** Consider the kind of day you're having and the capacity you have at present. For example, you decide that every Monday, Wednesday, and Friday you're going to do a resistance training workout, but it can be as short as five minutes. *Every second of self-care is significant.*

2 **You have a Plan A, B, and C:** To continue with the previous example, you plan to do your non-negotiable five-minute to one-hour workout at 5:30 a.m., before the rest of the world wakes up, but if you miss that, you can

pivot and do it before lunchtime. And if that doesn't work out, you can do it before dinner.

3. **Simple shifts help you maintain forward motion:** If a ship changes course by just one degree, over time it will arrive in a completely different location. Stay committed to consistency by doing *any* small thing to boost your wellbeing. For example, if you absolutely have to eat a midafternoon cookie, add a handful of nuts or a hunk of cheese to help stabilize your blood sugar.

When Pamela was on a fabulous tropical holiday in Maui, she applied the flexible framework to her long-distance running routine. "Usually, I find it hard to run on holidays because I can't imagine trying to figure out a twenty-kilometer route, but this morning I ran four kilometres, and I feel amazing!" she reported.

EMBRACE TYPE 2 FUN

Even if you adopt a flexible framework, what if you find it challenging to savour exercise, indulge in vegetables, and delight in early bedtimes? Here's a sneaky workaround. Human nature aims to move toward pleasure and away from pain, so it's important to be aware of how you define the healthy habits you wish to practice. Across the pleasure–pain spectrum there is

- *destructive pain*, which feels bad and is bad for you;
- *constructive pain*, which feels bad but is good for you;

- *destructive pleasure*, which feels good but is bad for you;
- *constructive pleasure*, which feels good and is good for you.

Constructive pleasure is a pretty easy one to comply with, like eating a handful of freshly picked strawberries on a beautiful summer day or relishing a big hug from someone you love. Let's zero in on constructive pain — also known as discomfort or Type 2 Fun.

Type 2 Fun is part of the Fun Scale, created by University of Alaska Fairbanks geology professor Rainer J. Newberry in the mid-eighties, which includes three types of fun:

- Type 1 Fun is fun in the moment.
- Type 2 Fun is fun only in retrospect.
- Type 3 Fun is miserable. Period.

Humans are efficient creatures who don't like to waste energy or be uncomfortable. As you learned in chapter 1, you can stay stuck when you are bumping up against the discomfort of an upper limit. You may shrink away from this discomfort without questioning its significance. Instead, you can rewire your brain to see discomfort — mental or physical — as an important stepping stone to a better life.

For example, my client Jane, a brand strategist and mom of a kindergartner, revolutionized the way she ate and moved. As she told me, "The fact that being uncomfortable — like being cold walking outside in the winter or eating vegetables when I don't want to — contributes to your life and longevity was mind-blowing to me and will always stick in my head. I have now learned to push through discomfort to get to the good part, which takes consistency because it gets easier to manage as you go."

I learned a lot about managing discomfort from my little brother, who introduced me to the concept of Type 2 Fun when he revealed how he encouraged his wife (who's a rugby-playing triathlete in her own right) to participate in some of his beloved, and extremely challenging, outdoor pursuits. At first, she may not have loved paddling through treacherous rapids or portaging through thick undergrowth, but as she and my brother reflected on their adventure from the comfort of their home, she sure felt amazing to have pushed herself to take part in such an incredible experience.

Type 2 Fun really resonated with me because retrospect — reviewing past events and reflecting on how they made me feel — was how I'd changed my behaviour and my brain (self-directed neuroplasticity for the win!). I began successfully applying this concept to wellbeing pursuits that I had previously found challenging to practice consistently.

Years later, I opened one of my multiday wellness retreats with this concept. I had worked in collaboration with the hotel's chef to provide decadent and nourishing gourmet meals, which were all included throughout the weekend, for our guests. On the last day, after completing modules on mindfulness, movement, nutrition, sleep, and connection, participants created a final action plan to take home, as a map to follow in this new phase of their life — as you'll do in chapter 10. One participant put up her hand. "I just had an aha moment," she said, after previously sharing with the group that eating healthfully, especially vegetables, was a very big challenge for her. "Salad is Type 2 Fun!" she declared. What an incredible mindset shift to transform her behaviour.

Discomfort is a major obstacle to personal growth and wellbeing, and may be at the root of some of the barriers to forward motion that you've encountered:

- **Busyness:** Do you feel like you need to fill your time being "productive"? Perhaps it's too uncomfortable to consider that you might need to grow your self-compassion, to allow yourself rest and recovery, and to stop putting your own needs last.

- **Time management:** Do you find yourself going down rabbit holes on social media, or saying yes to commitments you know you lack the capacity for? Is that because of the perceived effort you will need to be fully present and focus on your dreams?

- **Emotional numbing:** Are there some feelings you should be feeling to expand to the next level of your life? Does that feel too hard to do right now so instead you eat or drink or shop or gamble or (fill in the blank)?

- **Fear:** Are you afraid to fail? Or is your greatness what you're really afraid of? Either way, this discomfort feels unknown, scary, or icky, so you stay put.

There will always be obstacles in your way, but when you don't see them — when you aren't aware, conscious, or mindful of them — you can't move past them. Here are some simple ways to do this.

MONITOR YOUR THOUGHTS

Have you heard the term "metacognition"? It's just a fancy word to describe the way you think about how you think. When you get into the habit of noticing your thoughts and inquiring if they're constructive, helpful, or true — versus destructive, unhelpful, and false — you can begin to upgrade the quality of your inner dialogue. This can help you grow your self-compassion and self-trust, which are two skills critical to making positive changes. If you don't believe you deserve to break free from destructive patterns or trust yourself to take consistent action to change your behaviour, you will stay stuck.

When you witness a negative thought, such as *There isn't time to take care of myself today* or *I'll start exercising tomorrow even though I said I'd do it today*, and let your psyche absorb it, you reinforce those limiting beliefs. You also support catastrophic thinking, where you assume the worst about everything and get pulled into a downward spiral of adversity.

The key to preventing that downward spiral is when you notice a poor-quality thought, stop it midway through, and choose a better thought. Equally, when you have a high-quality thought, you can consciously choose to feel it more deeply to reinforce it, and then take action immediately before your limiting beliefs talk you out of it.

For example, when you have a moment of inspired thinking like *I should get out of bed now and go for a walk*, if you immediately move your body to action (instead of snoozing), you will add more time and energy to your day. Or if you think, *If I turn off my notifications for thirty minutes, I can start working on that book I've always dreamed of writing*, instead of getting sidetracked answering an endless queue of emails first, you will be prioritizing your dreams in doable chunks so you can consistently make progress and hardwire your brain to continue operating this way.

Again, this is all about making mindful choices that will benefit you so you can feel better right now!

DO LESS: A COUNTERINTUITIVE APPROACH TO HAVE MORE

Another tool to help you stay on track and consistently move forward is to reduce the amount of time you spend dividing your attention, what we call multitasking. It can be hard not to feel frazzled and scattered when you are wearing multiple hats and notifications are coming at you from every angle. Perhaps you're checking emails while watching TV or while eating dinner and reconnecting with your family after a long day. How can you have a better sense of connection and accomplishment in your work, family, and leisure life? By focusing on one thing at a time, otherwise known as *uni-tasking*.

Beyond diminishing our relationships, the costs of multitasking include decreased cognition and productivity, impaired decision-making, and activation of the stress response. "Each time we switch our attention from one thing to another, there's a metabolic cost — we use up neural resources," neuroscientist Daniel Levitin told me during an interview for an article I wrote about the art of uni-tasking. "After a bunch of switching in a short time span, we stress the system," he said. "This can cause cortisol, the stress hormone, to be released, which triggers the stress response, downgrading our immune, digestive, reproductive, and growth systems, mobilizing more energy to fight or flee. This, in turn, can cloud your thinking, and the irony is that you don't even realize your thinking has been clouded because it is too clouded to notice."

Sometimes we have no choice but to multitask. However, when you can safely and responsibly uni-task, you reduce your stress, increase your energy, magnify your productivity, and offer your full presence to those you love and care about. Levitin also made several suggestions that will help you make a deliberate effort to uni-task.

- **Unplug:** Exit the "novelty loop" that is social media, notifications, and news, and replace it with activities like yoga, exercise, meditation, music, and nature immersion. You can also try periodically unplugging by using a time management tool or method like the

Pomodoro Technique. With this approach, you turn off all distractions, set an alarm, and work for an uninterrupted period of time. This philosophy also applies to quality time with friends and family.

- **Download:** Write down everything you have to do. This clears your mind of clutter, relieves you from replaying your to-do list, and allows you to better focus on the task at hand.
- **Prioritize:** Rewrite your to-do list in order of importance so you don't get distracted from working on the tasks that are top priority.

Think of all the extra time you'll now have to be more focused, mindful, and aware! Take a moment to reinforce these concepts and harness the power of self-directed neuroplasticity by completing the exercise at the end of the chapter.

ONCE YOU'VE decided what's most important in your life, how do you keep moving forward with motivation and consistency? Hire a great coach! (Spoiler: it's you.)

TENETS OF FEELING BETTER: NEUROPLASTICITY

- Practice mindfulness: the state of being conscious, or aware, of how your thoughts, words, and actions make you feel.

- Choose self-directed neuroplasticity: the active, conscious process of brain rewiring.

- Use the flexible framework to banish the all-or-nothing mentality and embrace imperfection.

- Adopt grey-zone thinking by choosing habits that can expand or contract.

- Create Plans A, B, and C, and apply simple shifts to help you maintain forward motion.

- Embrace Type 2 Fun (also known as constructive pain, mild adversity, or discomfort).

- Focus on one thing at a time (uni-task) by unplugging, downloading, and prioritizing.

Consider the 3 As

1. **Ask:** What made you feel good (in practice and retrospect)? In your journal, write down three to seven things that answer this question.

2. **Affirm** the significance of constructive habits. In your journal, write down three or more benefits of practicing constructive habits.

3. **Act:** Practice, and reflect on, constructive habits in a flexible framework. In your journal, write down the actions required to feel good, then confirm that you've completed them and how that made you feel.

CHAPTER 4

The Magic Formula

*"Discipline means to be a disciple
of your true self that lies within."*
GURMUKH KAUR KHALSA

IMAGINE WHAT your life could look like if you had a great coach. Someone who supported your growth and championed your dreams by

- asking good questions,
- identifying goals,
- helping troubleshoot,
- offering encouragement,
- pinpointing efficiencies,
- providing accountability,
- building skills,
- developing strategies,
- presenting big-picture advice,
- facilitating insights.

What if that someone could be *you*? What if you could be in charge of your own momentum enhancement?

For most of my twenties, I worked as a full-time personal trainer. My goal was always to enable my clients to create their own programs by revealing the rationale behind each exercise, so they could stay motivated and consistent when we weren't training together. However, I came to understand, as I showed you earlier, that knowing doesn't equal doing.

How could I help motivate my clients to perpetually stoke their inner fire? This was something that I struggled with personally, and I couldn't show anyone the way until I'd taken the trip myself. When I reverse engineered my transformation, I revealed how to communicate safety to my nervous system (chapter 2) and how to rewire my brain to support habit formation and elimination (chapter 3). I also broke down the steps I'd been taking on a daily basis to fuel my forward motion.

Through the power of strategic repetition, I reprogrammed my mind (thoughts) and my brain (neural structure) to keep my determination steady. I realized those steps were a simple and cyclical formula, a template that anyone could easily follow. It worked so well it felt like magic, so I called it the Magic Formula.

The Magic Formula provides the perfect conditions to spark self-directed neuroplasticity and offers questions to keep you focused on exactly what you need to thrive. Asking good questions is the key skill of a great coach. Your brain is a problem-solving machine and will answer any question you ask it. This is why it's so important to know the difference between constructive questions and destructive questions.

Destructive questions usually begin with *why*, like "Why is this happening to me?" or "Why can't anything ever go my way?" It's best to avoid those defeating inquiries.

Constructive questions usually start with *how* and *what*, like "How can I shift this situation?" or "What can I do right now to feel better?" Focus on these empowering inquiries.

The Magic Formula is a self-coaching model to help you generate ongoing self-discovery, self-healing, and self-actualization through constructive questioning, guided reflection, and data collection. In this chapter, I will walk you through its five repeating steps:

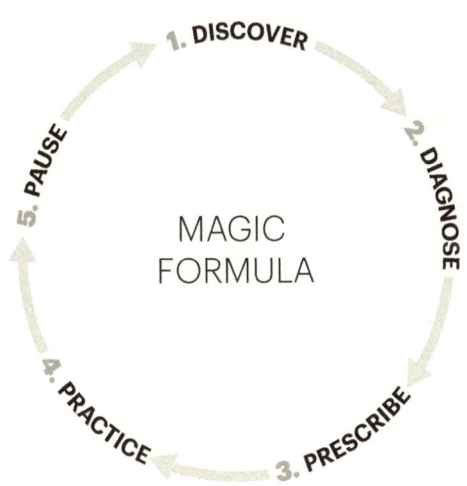

1. DISCOVER: BUILD YOUR INNER AND OUTER AWARENESS

In chapters 1, 2, and 3, you learned to ask great questions like

- What do I truly want?
- What do I need to feel safe?
- What habits do I want to build or break?

These are incredibly powerful questions to ponder every day, across every area of your life, because they help you become more mindful of how your thoughts, words, and actions are serving you. Constructive questions help you build inner awareness and outer awareness.

You are developing outer awareness right now as you read this book, and as you listen to podcasts, attend workshops, query experts, or engage in discussions with friends and colleagues. Whenever you hit a roadblock, you can ask yourself, "What resources can I seek to help me understand more?" And even better, you can tune in to your inner awareness by asking, "What do I already know to be true?"

Metacognition (thinking about how you think) is a tool of inner awareness. Applying mindset shifts is a metacognitive tool to help you think a little differently. Here are seven mindset shifts to help you build your inner awareness and blast through roadblocks by helping you form better questions.

1. Challenge Mindset

Studies show that simply thinking about your stress differently can change both your physiological and psychological response to it. You can strive to meet a challenge without the drastic spikes in cortisol and adrenaline, and with greater self-efficacy, when you feel a sense of connection and control. To engage this mindset, ask yourself questions like "What tools do I have to meet this challenge?" and "How can I rise to the occasion?"

2. Connection Mindset

As we are social beings, one of the most stressful beliefs we can hold is that we are alone or that we don't belong. To keep yourself moving forward, look for and open yourself to micro- and macro-moments of human connection. In her TED Talk "The Secret to Living Longer May Be Your Social Life," developmental psychologist Susan Pinker says that the greatest predictors of longevity are not your diet, weight, sleep, exercise, or marital status, but your close relationships and social integration — meaning how much human interaction you have in your day. To engage this mindset, ask yourself questions like "Where do I already have support?" and "How can I grow my sense of connection?"

3. Curiosity Mindset

When you can meet a challenge with an eagerness to understand it rather than with frustration, hopelessness, or shame, you can boost the resources you have to overcome it. To engage this mindset, ask yourself questions like "What is the deeper meaning here?" and "How can I find success in this situation?"

4. Good-Enough Mindset

How do you continue to banish the all-or-nothing mentality? By applying the good-enough mindset. To engage this mindset, ask yourself questions like "What actions can I be happy with while staying committed to consistency?" and "How can I shift my expectations to maintain forward motion?"

5. Growth Mindset

Believing that you can always continue to change, adapt, and grow is a powerful way to think. To engage this mindset, ask yourself questions like "What did I learn from this experience?" and "How can I do better next time?"

6. Positivity Mindset

As you learned in chapter 3, your brain's negativity bias is a force you must balance by consciously savouring good experiences, if you want to avoid getting stuck in patterns of negative rumination. I like to think of these two complementary forces as antennae: sensory devices scanning for both threats and blessings. Because negativity is so much stronger than positivity, a daily practice of scanning for good can be transformative. In his TED Talk "The Happy Secret to Better Work," happiness researcher Shawn Achor says, "If you can raise somebody's level of positivity in the present, then their brain experiences what we now call a 'happiness advantage.'... Your intelligence rises, your creativity rises, your energy levels rise. Your brain at positive is 31 per cent more productive than your brain at negative, neutral, or stressed."

Growing your positivity antennae can also help you overcome adversity. This was the case for my client Gisele, a motivational speaker and author, who, in the span of eighteen months, supported her husband through a heart attack and subsequent quadruple bypass heart surgery, suffered a devastating miscarriage, and grieved the sudden loss of both her parents and her father-in-law. "I think that most of my being able to stay sober for the last five years, while navigating so much grief, I owe to my gratitude practice," she said. "Every day at nine o'clock my Gratitude Alarm goes off and I practice gratitude, and I've been doing that since 2016 because of you. Now almost everyone in my life does it too. A few days before my mom died — just three weeks after learning she had pancreatic cancer — my sister flew in and the three of us practiced gratitude together. And then when my dad died, me, my aunt, my uncle, my grandma, and my sister all stood around him and we did gratitude together. I really believe that there's always something to be grateful for."

In addition to practicing gratitude, it's important to remember that our negativity bias is a crucial built-in safety mechanism, and that we need to acknowledge the nudges we receive about what needs to change. "In order to heal, it is essential to gather the strength to think negatively," says Gabor Maté in *When the Body Says No*. "Negative thinking... is a willingness to consider what is not working. What is not in balance? What have I ignored? What is my body saying no to? Without these questions, the stress responsible for our lack of balance will remain hidden."

To balance these two complementary forces in your life, try a practice I call Gratitude + Discontent by asking yourself questions like "What's good?" in addition to "What's not working?" Aim to make the former list at least two to three times as long as the latter.

7. Recovery Mindset

As you learned in chapter 2, it's critical to assemble a toolbox of practices that help you activate your parasympathetic nervous system and complete the stress cycle. To engage this mindset, ask yourself questions like "How can I make time for recovery today?" and "What somatic or cognitive tools can I use right now?"

2. DIAGNOSE: IDENTIFY ISSUES — BOUNDARIES AND BARRIERS

You can't move past a barrier if you can't even see that it's in your way. So it's helpful to run through a daily shortlist of diagnostic questions to address and resolve potential obstructions.

- Is there an *inner barrier*, such as a limiting belief that's preventing you from taking a bold step forward?

- Or is it an *outer barrier*, such as forgetting to set your workout clothes aside last night and now you're at risk of missing your workout because you don't want to wake your family by gathering the items you need?

- To *identify* and *rectify* barriers, ask yourself questions like "What are the issues I'm struggling with?" and "How can I remove this barrier?"

It's also imperative to protect your passage on the freeway to success by installing boundaries to keep your path clear.

- First, consider your *inner boundaries*, the commitments you've made to yourself, the operational standards you hold, the discipline you're devoted to.

- Next, which *outer boundaries* do you already have in place? Is your family aware of your self-care schedule? Do you advertise and implement office hours?

- To *create* and *state* boundaries, ask yourself questions like "What am I committed to practicing?"; "How can I stay true to my standards today?"; "Have I clearly shared my boundaries with the community I engage with?"; and "What do I need to add or remove to feel successful?"

As you build your toolkit of constructive questions, you can gain so much momentum when you use them in concert, like my client Yvonne. She is a marketing executive who was struggling to strike a better balance between the complex care her son, who uses a wheelchair, needed, and the sleep, exercise, and reflection time she needed to feel her best but wasn't getting.

Yvonne used the curiosity mindset to discover how she could find success in these areas of her life and diagnosed that she could install boundaries around her morning and evening practices by removing a barrier for her son. Because he has limited use of his limbs, he needs her help with his bedtime routine. But because he's a smart young man with curiosities of his own to pursue, he likes to stay up late, so Yvonne was chronically sleep deprived. For her, the answer to creating better balance came in three parts:

- She completed her role in his bedtime routine earlier in the evening and installed an iPad mount on his wheelchair, so he had independence to read and have access to programs.

- She created wind-down time for herself by letting her inner circle know she turns her phone off at 8:00 p.m. This allowed Yvonne to calm her mind, journal, and practice gratitude, so she always hit that headspace when she was going to bed.

- She purchased a Peloton bike so that she could exercise at home early in the morning (which she was then well-rested enough to do) before her son woke up.

3. PRESCRIBE: CREATE A SCHEDULED AND FLEXIBLE PLAN

To get clear on your doable and delicious plan, ask yourself questions like "Where can I insert the healthy habits I intend to practice?" and "What habits will serve me best given the time and tools I currently have?"

- **Block out time** in your calendar to create a scheduled yet flexible plan. You may discover that in order to say yes to your wellbeing, you may have to say no to the requests of others.

- **Create short scripts** to simplify the often tricky process of saying no, like "Apologies, I'm currently at capacity" or "Sorry, my schedule is full." Notice these do not include details of why you're unavailable or future promises to deliver.

4. PRACTICE: TAKE ACTION WITH COMMITMENT AND CURIOSITY

Here's where we shift from knowing to doing — by taking action. It sounds silly when you really think about it, but this is the step where many of us stall. We've gathered all the information we need, built awareness around its importance, even invested in super cute workout clothes, but something prevents us from following through on our plans. This is why you need to stay deeply connected to what you truly want and committed to creating the life you dream is possible.

I've made a list of non-negotiable practices that help me align with my best self and posted multiple copies of it around my home and office, so that I'm reminded of the actions I intend to take every day. Here's how to do that for yourself:

- Reignite and reaffirm your commitment with questions like "What are the short-term and long-term benefits I'm about to experience?" and "How will these practices help me show up with integrity for the incredible person I know myself to be?"

- When you feel your motivation waning, get curious and ask yourself questions like "How could this tension, tiredness, or resistance be improved by a few micro-practices?"

- Set your mind into problem-solving mode by asking the question "How will I take action today?"

Another tool to fuel action with commitment and curiosity is to develop a personal mantra.

When I was an adult, my mom reminded me of my childhood mantra: "That's impossible, I can do that!" I loved this idea so much that I wrote it across the top of my vision board in bold, gold letters. Or you could borrow the fabulous Ultimate Success Mantra from *The Big Leap* by Gay Hendricks: "I expand in abundance, success, and love every day, as I inspire those around me to do the same," which will get you to asking, "How can I expand in abundance, success, and love today?" or "What can I do (despite its impossibility)?"

5. PAUSE: EXAMINE THE RESULTS OF YOUR ACTIONS

Pausing to reflect is *the* most important step of the Magic Formula. Even if you didn't take action, reflecting on how lousy neglecting your wellbeing made you feel can motivate you to make better choices from this moment on. You can examine the results of your actions — constructive or destructive — by asking questions like "How did that make me feel?" and "What could I have done to make myself feel better?"

This step is an important process of gathering data to confirm your hypothesis that self-care is a worthy investment of your time. Armed with empirical evidence that applies directly to your own life, you can see the unequivocal proof that your wellbeing really does matter and can be tended to in this easy-breezy, flexible framework.

This process of strategic repetition — learning, thinking, writing, speaking, rereading, sharing, practicing, and reassessing — sparks self-directed neuroplasticity and hardwires constructive thoughts, and actions, into your brain. You will suddenly find yourself thinking wonderful thoughts, such as *I'm feeling a little overwhelmed and will now go for a short nature walk to help manage my stress!* instead of *I will now devour this bag of vending machine junk along with my tenth coffee of the day!* It takes just ten to thirty seconds to begin the process of rewiring your brain, and when you write down the insights that arise when you pause, you magnify the power of these structural changes.

In addition to examining results, make time to re-examine your objectives. Do your dreams and goals still

Learn, think, write, speak, reread, share, practice, reassess.

---

feel like a good fit? Also make time to connect with your future vision: What does your life look like — and feel like — when you've already achieved your goals and are living your dreams?

Picture yourself having taken consistent, constructive actions. What do you see? How does it feel to have what you truly want? I will walk you through an incredible tool to do this on a much deeper level in chapter 9, but in the meantime, make time every day — even just thirty seconds — to close your eyes and connect with the vision you have for your life and reinforce the practices you've already gained to achieve that reality.

NEVER DOUBT this: you have everything you need inside of you to be your own great coach.

To fully support your growth and champion your dreams, you will need discipline. If that is not a word you like to use, consider my definition: Discipline is the commitment to becoming the vision you have of your future self. It's the practice of behaving in alignment with a defined set of standards. And those standards are your wellness prescription — your micro-manifesto — which you'll develop and finesse in chapter 10.

Now it's time to learn the rituals that will complete the curriculum you need to finish writing your wellness prescription. Are you ready? Let's go!

TENETS OF FEELING BETTER: SELF-COACHING

- **Discover:** Build awareness — inner and outer
- **Diagnose:** Identify issues — boundaries and barriers
- **Prescribe:** Create a plan — scheduled and flexible
- **Practice:** Take action — committed and curious
- **Pause:** Review results — spark neuroplasticity and revisit objectives

Consider the 3 As

1. **Ask:** What do I know? (Discover); What do I need? (Diagnose); What do I do? (Prescribe); How will I practice? (Practice); How did that feel? (Pause). In your journal, choose a challenge you have right now and write down the answer to each of the questions above.

2. **Affirm** the significance of your efforts as your own coach. In your journal, write down three or more benefits of being your own great coach.

3. **Act:** Practice, and reflect on, the Magic Formula daily. In your journal, write down the formula's five steps, then confirm how it made you feel to apply these steps to a challenge.

3
THE RITUALS

A deeply sincere set of habits practiced according to a prescribed order

CHAPTER 5

Move Your Body

*"Exercise is the most transformative
thing you can do for your brain."*
WENDY SUZUKI

DURING MY darkest days, all I wanted was a sense of hope. I wanted to believe that things could get better, but I didn't. I felt powerless, hopeless, and depressed. But then I learned that I had the power to rescue myself, revolt against the oppressive forces holding me down, and take control of my life. I want you to know that, right now, you have that power too.

The sense of hope I began to develop came from a surprising place: my body.

Through conscious connection with my body, beginning with that delicious, sunny moment on my patio, the lens I was looking through changed, which meant that I was also changing my brain, for the better. As I developed the ability to be deeply rooted in mindfulness, I felt tendrils of hope reaching out to me. With practice, my grip on hope grew stronger and stronger. I could feel my dreams being born.

Since then, I've had a little notebook that I call the Dream Book, and every December 31 my husband and I fill in one page, alternating lines with our individual and collective goals for the twelve months ahead. I transcribe that list to a larger piece of paper and post it in the middle of the corkboard next to my desk so that I have daily reminders of the life I intend to create.

For years now, my primary goal has been to move, meditate, and reflect every day to feel happy, hopeful, and strong. It's a simple directive that's incredibly powerful because it lays the foundation for my overall wellbeing. I covered reflection in the last chapter in step 5 of the Magic Formula, and I will talk more about meditation in chapter 9. In this chapter, I want to share my six-part definition of movement:

1. Physical activity: how much you move throughout the day
2. Breath: how you breathe
3. Posture: the expansiveness and alignment of your body
4. Strength: the quality of your skeletal muscle
5. Endurance: the health of your heart and lungs
6. Mobility: the range of motion in your joints

Don't despair if this sounds like a lot. It's quite simple to weave multifaceted movement throughout your day when you step back to consciously design it. My morning ritual alone checks five of the six movement areas above and often takes less than twenty minutes.

You may find that your primary catalyst is different, but for me it's my morning ritual of move-meditate-reflect that sets the stage for the other rituals that I will talk about in the next three chapters — nourishment, rest, and connection — to fall into place. If you move your body first thing in the morning, you are much more likely to make positive dietary choices; prioritize your rest and bedtime rituals; and be more open, present, and compassionate in the multitude of relationships in your life.

MOVE MORE, FEEL BETTER: THE ANTI-SEDENTARY REVOLUTION

For me, everyday wellness begins with the decision to move upon waking. That daily decision — that discipline — is a big part of my commitment to what I call the anti-sedentary revolution. My wild nature needs me to be physically active. And so does yours.

Humans have been around for hundreds of thousands of years, but it's been only in the last one hundred (only a tiny fraction of a single percentage point of our existence) that our lives have become dangerously sedentary. We evolved as highly active creatures, and our body — from our cardiovascular, respiratory, and digestive systems to our reproductive, lymphatic, and nervous systems — still needs us to operate as such.

The anti-sedentary revolution was my response to learning about sedentary physiology. The impact of *inactivity* is so different from the benefits of *activity* that scientists had to create a whole new field of study! Low-energy expenditure activities aren't neutral — they're detrimental. Being inactive doesn't just cause you to miss out on the myriad benefits of movement, it also introduces a whole lot of unnecessary suffering to your life. Even when you do get adequate exercise, sedentary behaviour is still bad for your mental and physical health.

According to the Sedentary Behaviour Research Network, "recent evidence suggests that having a high level of sedentary behaviour negatively impacts health independent of other factors including body weight, diet, and physical activity." This is what is meant by the adage "Sitting is the new smoking." And research points to anxiety, depression, and other mental disorders as being inversely proportional to physical activity. The less you move, the worse you feel — inside and out.

Sedentary physiology looks at the body functions upset by inactivity, whereas exercise physiology looks at the body functions that thrive via activity. I have long been singing the praises of exercise — I've been a certified fitness instructor, personal trainer, and older adult specialist for more than twenty years — but I initially thought that once I'd checked a resistance, endurance, or mobility workout off the list, I could expect vibrant health throughout the rest of the day. Turns out that isn't true. Even if you hit the gym for an hour every single day before driving home, sitting down to eat, parking yourself at the computer to work, getting lost in a scroll-fest with your handheld device, then relaxing in front of the TV before going to sleep, you're still spending twenty-three hours of your day inactive. That's 96 per cent of your life.

"We are designed to be wild, and by living tamely we make ourselves sick and unhappy," says Harvard Medical School psychiatry professor John J. Ratey in *Go Wild*. "Sedentary behaviour causes brain impairment, and we know how: by depriving your brain of the flood of neurochemistry that evolution developed in order to grow brains and keep them healthy."

Before we became so tame, we had to move to stay alive. But now here we are, sitting around all day, slouched over, pressing buttons, and ordering ready-made food straight to our plates (that a machine then cleans) instead of travelling many miles to find the ingredients for our sustenance. These days, we have to move to *thrive*. We must consciously choose to provide the flood of neurochemistry that our brains need to function well. You can rewild by joining the anti-sedentary revolution.

"Movement places demands on the brain, just as it does on muscle, and so the brain releases BDNF [brain-derived neurotrophic factor], which triggers the growth of [brain] cells to meet the increased mental demands of movement. But BDNF floods throughout the brain, not just to the parts engaged in movement. Thus, the whole brain flourishes as a result of movement," says Ratey.

This movement-induced flood of neurochemistry is delivered by your cardiovascular system thanks to your heart and lungs. Here's a fun fact: of your body's approximately thirty trillion cells, twenty-five trillion of them are red blood cells. That's 83 per cent of the cells in your body working nonstop to deliver oxygen to the remaining 17 per cent of your cells. And while only 2 per cent of your body weight, your brain requires up to 25 per cent of the oxygen you breathe and energy you consume. But movement doesn't just help fuel your brain with oxygen, it also changes it.

7 Exciting Benefits of Physical Activity

Movement sparks neuroplasticity (the rewiring of brain cells) and neurogenesis (the birth of new brain cells), making *every kind of lifestyle change* that much easier. With movement, you are not only forging important new connections, but also recruiting new brain cells to support the campaign. These positive changes provide the following benefits:

1 Movement improves learning, memory, and other cognitive functions, such as problem-solving, decision-making, and attention.

2 Movement protects the brain from mood and cognitive disorders, such as anxiety, depression, and dementia.

3 Movement combats the detrimental effects of stress, helping you complete the stress cycle, by metabolizing excess cortisol and blood sugar, and become more resilient in the face of future stresses.

4 Movement expands your self-trust and confidence, making you more likely to see opportunities and seize them.

5. Movement manufactures a delicious cocktail of feel-good chemicals (like serotonin, dopamine, oxytocin, endorphins, and endocannabinoids) that increase your joy, enjoyment, and courage.

6. Movement primes us for social connection, downregulating our hypervigilance to psychological threats, increasing our sense of belonging, and helping us combat loneliness.

7. Movement changes our microbiome for the better, improving the diversity and strength of the helpful microbes in our gut.

I mean, come on, that's incredible! No drugs can match the power of movement to provide these benefits. And please remember, we're talking about just *minutes*, here and there. It's so doable. But wait, there's more!

Physical activity provides all of these benefits — and exercise amplifies them.

"In the wild, regular exercise helped clear stress-based cortisol out of the body, but our sedentary lifestyle allows cortisol to keep circulating, which increases reactivity in a vicious circle," says Rick Hanson. Daily movement rituals allow us to be more responsive and less reactive — what a beautiful gift to our life and relationships.

The Snack Method

A motivating visual that always inspires me to move is to think of maintaining my circulatory system as a bright, babbling brook — versus the stinky, stagnant pond of sedentarism. Eww. The rewards of doing this are many, and the costs are so small that even *one minute* has an impact on your psychological and physical wellbeing.

I use the snack method to make sure I get enough physical activity during my workday. I set a timer in increments of twenty-five to seventy-five minutes (remember the Pomodoro Technique from chapter 3?), and when it goes off, I have to move for at least one minute. This practice has the added benefit of helping me stay focused on the task at hand, as I generally turn off all notifications while the timer is running (uni-tasking for the win!). Here are some suggestions to keep your brook babbling:

- Morning and midday mini-workouts: See more below.

- Housework: Do the dishes, make the bed, or sweep the floor.

- Collaboration: Encourage "moving meetings" at the office by scheduling walk-and-talks.

- Connection: Instead of meeting for coffee or cocktails, suggest physically active dates with friends and family, such as a hike or bike ride.

- Afternoon delight: Yep, I'm suggesting *that* kind of quickie.

The snack method can help you weave movement into your daily life, but it's important to make sure your environment isn't working against you.

Set Up Your Environment

It's not just dementia, cancers, cardiovascular and inflammatory diseases (like bowel disease, asthma, and rheumatoid arthritis), and infectious agents (like viruses and bacteria) that can flourish when you're inactive. Negative mental states and disorders (like depression, anxiety, rumination, and even self-criticism) can flourish too. To make it much easier to weave physical activity into your day, set yourself up for success with these suggestions to upgrade your environment.

Design your home to inspire movement: While writing this chapter, I went out for a midday walk and noticed an interesting scene through someone's living room window: a row of exercise equipment in front of the TV, instead of a couch! In my own home, I've sprinkled different kinds of exercise equipment all over, including a chin-up bar and gymnastics rings in my home office, kettlebells in my living/dining room, resistance bands and yoga mats in my bedroom, and a home gym in my basement — so I'm encouraged to do a little bit of movement at every turn.

Design your social life around physical activity: Add more active dates to your calendar — and novelty to your life — by trying new physical adventures with friends, such as an after-work paddleboard or a cross-country ski, or a weekend hike or tennis match. As mentioned above, exercise primes your brain for connection and diminishes the negative effects of stress, so all of your relationships will benefit from being active together.

Design your life around active transportation: Use your body to get places. Walk, bike (or row your boat) to school, work, and extracurricular activities, and to run errands. I cannot get over the missed opportunity for some much-needed physical activity in my own neighborhood, where a staggering number of children who attend schools that are within a ten- to thirty-minute walk away are driven there each morning, before they're forced to sit still for much of the day. I recognize that many parents are on their way to work, to which they must drive, and this points to larger issues of walkability, work-life balance, and busyness. We need a complete restructuring of society to better support wellbeing and longevity, but that's a bigger conversation for another day.

Honouring Children's Right to Move

Young children are deeply connected to their basic instinct to move and should be given the freedom to satisfy this desire. Their physical and psychological health also suffers when we force them to be inactive, contained in carriers, baby seats, strollers, or at desks, for much of the day.

We must keep our children wild by strengthening — not hindering — their motivation to move their growing bodies. Just as I prioritize my own movement, I see it as my parental responsibility to provide movement opportunities for my child. Once my daughter learned to walk, we mostly ditched the stroller, so she could build her physical abilities and join us in the anti-sedentary revolution.

Although this practice means it takes you longer to get places (toddlers toddle!) and requires greater patience, it is well worth the cost: you will be setting them up for a lifetime of attuning to and honouring their body's needs.

Plus, family adventures that include movement help build stronger bonds. From the time my daughter was eighteen months, we've ventured with her on weekend excursions of at least five kilometres, often to our local bakery for sourdough bread, or to the reward of a waterfront brunch after a hike in the forest. And since she was three years old, we've used our tandem bike to do errands, such as exchange backpacks loaded with books at the library or fill them with goodies from the local farmers' market.

BEFORE I explain exercise in greater detail, let's take a look at the influence of your breath and posture on how you feel. These two things are fundamental to every kind of movement, whether that's daily physical activity or exercises to develop your strength, endurance, and mobility. Shallow breathing and misaligned posture are the enemies of good circulation, and can create unwanted stress and increase your chances of injury.

BREATH

Breathwork has become a popular practice, but what does that term even mean? I use the following terms interchangeably because they all involve manipulating your breath on purpose: breathwork, mindful breathing, conscious breathing, deep breathing, and diaphragmatic breathing. Why is breathwork important in helping you feel better? Because it has a huge impact on your nervous and circulatory systems.

Shallow breathing is both an *activator* of the sympathetic nervous system and a *sign* of sympathetic nervous system activation. Remember the cascade of nonideal things that happen when you're chronically stressed that I listed in chapter 2? Paying attention to your breath is an easy way to reduce your overall stress load.

There's a phenomenon called "screen apnea" where your level of stimulation from staring at emails or scrolling through social media causes you to breathe irregularly and even cease breathing for longer than optimal. That irregular breathing alerts your brain that something is wrong and activates the fight-or-flight response, which is marked by rapid, shallow breathing to temporarily increase oxygen consumption.

Do you catch yourself sighing often? That's your body rebelling against a stress-induced tendency to hold your breath or breathe shallowly. Enter my absolute favourite muscle in the body: the diaphragm — a marvellous muscle regulated by both the somatic and autonomic nervous systems. It functions both unconsciously (working hard 24-7) and consciously (stop reading for a second and take a big, deep breath).

Mindful breathing is the deliberate contraction and expansion of your diaphragm, and there are exercises you can do to help maximize this muscle. Remember the body-based, bottom-up, somatic tools from chapter 2? The following exercise is one of my favourites.

1-2-3 Breathing

I teach a technique that I call 1-2-3 Breathing. This easy practice has the quadruple whammy of activating your parasympathetic nervous system, strengthening your respiratory muscles, increasing your lung capacity, and expanding your posture. Plus, when used as the point of focus during meditation, which is what I do most days, it has the added benefit of improving your ability to be present. Here's how to do it.

As you inhale: Imagine your torso as a three-dimensional box that's expanding in width, depth, and height. If you need proprioceptive feedback, try sitting upright in a hard-back chair with your hands on either side of your ribs, fingers wrapped around your front and thumbs wrapped around your back.

1. Expand the depth of your ribs so they swell forward and press backward into the chair.

2. Expand the width of your ribs so they push out into your hands.

3. Expand the height of your torso so that your ribs lift and separate between your hands, without letting them flare forward.

Inhale fully; see what's possible. Don't be afraid of this expansiveness. It's okay if it feels weird to allow your tummy to relax. A Harvard Health Publishing article says that "body image has a negative impact on respiration in our culture" because so many people hold in their stomachs, which "interferes with deep breathing, increases tension and anxiety, and limits the diaphragm's range of motion."

As you exhale: Stay where you are (in your chair, with your hands on your ribs) and imagine your torso as a three-dimensional box that's shrinking in width, depth, and height.

1 Contract and lift your pelvic floor muscles. Imagine the highly webbed, figure-eight-shaped group of muscles that support your bladder and bowels (and uterus, if you have one) shrinking and elevating, and firmly hold it there for the remainder of your exhale.

2 Shrink-wrap your transversus abdominis (TVA) in 360 degrees, like a corset tightening — try poking yourself on the side of your stomach while exhaling with a loud F sound if you're having trouble locating this muscle.

3 Shrink-wrap your ribs so that the tips of both your fingers and thumbs move toward each other.

Exhale fully; let it go. Bonus points if you can make your exhale longer than your inhale, as this activates the parasympathetic nervous system, via the vagus nerve, and helps elicit the recovery response.

One last note: most of your breathing should be through your nose. Inhaling through your nose humidifies, heats, and helps filter the air of pollutants, viruses, and bacteria — plus, studies suggest that nose breathing can even have a regulating effect on your nervous system.

Exhaling through your nose can prevent nasal dryness, strengthen respiratory muscles, increase lung capacity, and actually change the shape of your face! (Check out James Nestor's fascinating book *Breath* to learn many more interesting things about your breath.)

POSTURE

Misaligned, contracted posture impacts every one of your body's systems and can lead to increased stress and anxiety, decreased focus and energy, mechanical disadvantage, and suboptimal organ function. So it's important to be mindful of your expansiveness and alignment, whether you're sitting, standing, or moving, and to be aware that the costs of spinal compression reach beyond your *physical* body to your *psychology*.

"Expanding your body language — through posture, movement, and speech — makes you feel more confident and powerful, less anxious and self-absorbed, and generally more positive," writes social psychologist Amy Cuddy (who shot to fame following her TED Talk on "power posing") in *Presence*.

We behave differently when we *feel* powerful. Power is the ability to effect change, within us and in the world around us. A sense of personal power not only gives you more hope for the future, but also helps you *create* a better future. Power, says Cuddy, activates a psychological and behavioural *approach* system, whereas powerlessness activates a psychological and behavioural *inhibition* system.

When we feel powerful, we have more motivation to achieve our goals, increased resistance to constraining cultural rules, greater immunity to limiting beliefs, and the psychic freedom to pursue our creative interests without inhibition. We become renegades, radicals, buoyant, galvanized to act.

When we feel powerless, we become crippled by inaction, anxious, increasingly attuned to psychological threats, and more likely to conform to social pressures. We become smaller, weighed down, and uninspired.

So many of our daily tasks and habits contract us physically, which then contracts our life. We humans work best when we're in motion, expansive, and in alignment — mentally, physically, and spiritually. You are a glorious human, I am certain of this, and you must take up more space. But you can't take up more space if you're compressed and out of alignment.

You can counteract compression and train yourself to take up more space by upgrading the way you do the following:

- **Think and speak about yourself:** Instantly stop self-criticism and limiting beliefs when you notice their presence and reframe your inner dialogue with love, compassion, and generosity.

- **Hold your body:** A great cue to reset your alignment is to imagine stacking the roof of your mouth over the crown of your heart. This instantly inspires you to lift your chest and retract your chin.

- **Strengthen your body:** You can liberate yourself from the oppressive force of powerlessness by building a body that is strong enough to hold itself expansively throughout the day, whether you are sitting or standing, active or inactive.

A sense of power — both physical and psychological — energizes us to make positive changes. When you feel powerful, you become a force for good. This is one of many good reasons to build a powerful body through resistance training. Resistance training, also referred to as strength training, introduces an opposing force to your muscles, in the form of body weight, bands, cables, dumbbells — even canned foods, small pets, or children — which causes them to improve in strength, size, and/or endurance (depending on the frequency, intensity, length, and type of training).

STRENGTH

When I began resistance training for high school basketball, I noticed that all the women were on the cardio side of the gym and all the men were on the weights side. This perplexing imbalance is part of the reason I became a personal trainer. Research suggests that we should be as concerned with increasing muscle mass as we are with decreasing fat mass when it comes to health metrics. I've never liked using the body mass index (BMI) as a guide with clients, as it takes only height and weight into account — and doesn't distinguish between muscle mass versus fat mass. When I was powerlifting in my late twenties, I put on a lot of muscle and clocked in at around 160 pounds (I'm five feet and nine inches tall), which put me on the border of the BMI's "overweight" rating.

I knew better than to feel bad about that number, but I worried how that metric might add to the absurd mindset that women should be as light and little as possible, and thus keep them from learning how to build powerful bodies. Many of my female clients express their concerns to me about bulking up when resistance training. But honestly, this is the absolute least of your worries, because it takes a massive level of commitment to "she-hulk" yourself.

Instead, increasing your skeletal muscle index (SMI) should be the priority for everyone.

SMI Is the New BMI

Why should you care about increasing your SMI? Because it's much easier to maintain muscle than build it, and while it's never too late to start, the younger you begin, the better — and the longer you will benefit from the incredible physical and psychological perks of having strong, healthy muscles (more on this below). After the age of thirty, muscle mass decreases by around 5 per cent per decade; this accelerates to around 10 per cent after age fifty. Thanks to the hormonal changes associated with menopause, women especially need to be serious about muscle mass to protect their bones from osteoporosis and steady their balance. Fractures in older age often don't have good outcomes.

So how do you measure your SMI? You don't, unless you have a fancy machine. Grip strength, however, has been shown to be a good measure of muscle mass. Head to your nearest playground and hit the monkey bars. If you can hang for a minute or more, you can give yourself a pat on the back. Another completely non-scientific way to determine your SMI at home is to flex your leg and arm muscles, give them a good feel, and measure how impressed you are with their solidity.

Here are a few more reasons to make sure you are building and maintaining your skeletal muscle.

1. **Skeletal muscle is responsible for up to 90 per cent of postprandial glucose uptake.** After you eat (the postprandial phase), your body breaks down the food and shuttles nutrients to where they're needed. It's only when there's an excess of those components circulating in your bloodstream that your wellbeing suffers. With adequate muscle mass, your body can excel at glucose homeostasis (blood sugar regulation), protecting you from metabolic diseases, and even slowing down the aging process.

2. **Skeletal muscle is the second-largest endocrine organ in your body.** When you move, your skeletal muscles secrete bioactive peptides called myokines that have far-reaching anti-inflammatory, metabolic, and regulatory effects throughout the brain and body. There are six hundred different kinds of myokines but here are three you should know about:

- Muscle-derived BDNF: This champion of neuroplasticity and neurogenesis enhances any kind of behaviour change (and isn't just produced in the brain).

- Insulin-like Growth Factor 1 (IGF-1) plays an important role in fat metabolism and regulates growth hormone — also known as the "fountain of youth."

- Irisin helps you burn body fat as fuel and has antidepressant and neuroprotective effects.

In case you are curious about the largest endocrine organ in the body, it's white adipose tissue. Your body fat secretes bioactive peptides too. You won't often hear me mention weight loss, but this is one great reason to be mindful of your fat mass, specifically your visceral fat (which surrounds your vital organs) — also known as "active fat" or "toxic fat" — because too much of it can be bad for your wellbeing. And while we're at it, waist circumference, which suggests not just your overall adipose tissue volume but specifically your visceral fat, is a much better measurement than BMI for assessing your fat mass.

3 **Skeletal muscle deficiency predicts the risk of all-cause mortality.** The less muscle you have, the shorter your life expectancy and the lesser your life quality. An article in the journal *Gerontology* reports that "elderly individuals with sarcopenia [low muscle mass and function] are more likely to suffer from cognitive decline, cognitive impairment, and other brain-related diseases."

But it's not just the elderly. Thanks to reduced physical activity and increased sedentary behaviour, sarcopenia is no longer a disease of old age. Young people are now at serious risk too. As we age, independence becomes exceedingly important, and muscular strength is critical to activities of daily living. I've seen this first-hand, from my volunteer days at a long-term care facility and from my work as the social and fitness director at a retirement residence. I want to be able to tie my own shoes and brush my own hair for as long as possible. Don't you?

To feel powerful enough to make the changes we want in our lives — over the length of our lifetime — we need to have not just the strength but also the stamina and flexibility to sustain forward motion.

ENDURANCE

Endurance training builds stamina by strengthening your heart and lungs. Any kind of aerobic activity such as running, cycling, canoeing, surfing, martial arts, yardwork, housework, dancing, and sexual activity will help build your endurance. But walking is one of the best endurance activities you can do for your wellbeing. It's good for your heart, lungs, brain, mind, and basically every part of your body. It's simple, free, gets you places, and provides you the opportunity to commune with nature. And you can easily modify your walk by changing your speed, terrain, or incline.

A regular walk (and other endurance activities along the intensity spectrum) will not only boost your physical health but can also increase your happiness. And here's one more fun fact: your gait speed has been dubbed the "sixth vital sign" because it's a good indicator of overall health. So please always stop to smell the roses, but then resume your effort!

MOBILITY

Mobility training is the practice of helping your body move freely, which requires flexibility, range of motion, and joint integrity. Whether you stretch your chest by holding a double high-five in your doorway before sitting down at your desk, or practice yoga, tai chi, Pilates, or other activities that elongate your muscles and lubricate your joints, stretching your body is an important daily habit to counteract compression, expand personal power, reduce tension, increase energy, reduce injury risk, and help you maintain independence with activities of daily living in later years.

The slow, repetitive movements and intentional breathing practices characteristic of many types of mobility training (and some types of endurance training) have the added benefit of providing the perfect environment for active meditation — a space for mindful awareness, inner noticing, and self-discovery.

CRAFTING YOUR OWN PROGRAM

The exercise guidelines I share with you in this chapter are designed to support your functional fitness, which is your ability to perform activities of daily living throughout your life. Beyond functional fitness, the movement rituals you will create for yourself — and the discipline necessary to practice them — will support your sense of personal power. This is the path to feeling better.

It's good to consistently challenge yourself, to reveal your competence. This takes embracing Type 2 Fun and seeing discomfort as advantageous. "Physical accomplishments can change how you think about yourself and what you are capable of," says health psychologist Kelly McGonigal in her book *The Joy of Movement*. "And once you've sensed yourself as powerful, it changes the way you look at an obstacle in your way."

It's also good to consider what you are training for. You can see your obstacles only when you know exactly where you're going — when you're clear on your goals. If you're training for a specific athletic event, you'll want to customize your training accordingly. In the pages of this book, the "event" we're training for is feeling better every day — expanding our capacity for joy, vitality, and abundance. For example, I am training to be a kind, compassionate, and fun mom, friend, and wife; to be a deeply present coach who can access my knowledge to maximize my clients' success; and to join the centenarian club so I can meet my grandkids, dance at their weddings, and pick up their kids.

As you create your own training program — with a blend of resistance, endurance, and mobility exercises — remember to use the flexible framework that I described in chapter 3, where habits, *rituals*, can expand or contract as needed. That said, my recommendations are that you aim for the following:

- Over three movement snacks per day (one to twenty minutes)
- Over five movement meals per week (twenty to sixty minutes)
- Over three movement feasts per month (over an hour)

Also consider:

- engaging a range of intensities from low-energy expenditure to high-energy expenditure activities;
- leaving at least one day between resistance training workouts (to aid muscle recovery) and high-impact endurance workouts, such as running (to protect your joints from overuse);
- including a variety of home workouts, travel workouts, community workouts, and nature workouts (also called "green exercise" — more on this in chapter 8) that focus on resistance, endurance, and mobility — separately or in combination.

Here's an example of my weekly exercise schedule:

- **Monday:** 10-to-45-minute resistance training and mobility training (plus a 15-minute walk, jog, or bike to and from school drop-off and pickup every weekday)
- **Tuesday:** 10-to-45-minute swim and mobility training
- **Wednesday:** 10-to-45-minute resistance training and mobility training
- **Thursday:** 10-to-45-minute run and mobility training
- **Friday:** 10-to-45-minute resistance training and mobility training
- **Saturday:** 10-to-45-minute bike and mobility training, plus a 60-to-120-minute family hike
- **Sunday:** 60-to-120-minute family hike

Now let's look at the specifics so you can create your own exercise program. With every exercise, be sure to always work within your capacity, build slowly and gradually, practice each movement with rapt focus and control, and consult an expert first if you are recovering from any injuries or limitations.

Resistance Training

If you want the most powerful and efficient resistance training workout, be sure to incorporate two types of activities: posterior-chain exercises and multi-muscle exercises.

Posterior-chain exercises strengthen the back of the body, counteracting poor posture and enabling you to carry yourself expansively. Many people with the best intentions — and already poor posture as a result of too much time in forward flexion (looking at a mobile device, sitting at the computer, slumped on the couch, or driving) — begin an exercise program only to magnify the compression they're experiencing by focusing on too many anterior-chain exercises, which strengthen the front of the body (like a bench press), and not enough posterior-chain exercises.

Examples of posterior-chain exercises include squats, lunges, dead lifts, rows, pull-ups, and pull-downs. When you are creating a workout to improve your posture and counteract compression, choose posterior-chain exercises in a two-, three-, or four-to-one ratio to anterior-chain exercises. This might sound complicated, but here is an example of what that might look like: two sets of a three-exercise kettlebell circuit that includes two posterior-chain exercises (squats and one-arm rows) and one anterior-chain exercise (chest press).

Multi-muscle exercises use multiple muscle groups and include all of the aforementioned exercises. These kinds of exercises give you the most bang for your buck because you're expanding the myriad benefits gained via muscular contraction (cognitive, metabolic, circulatory, endocrine) when you recruit more muscles at a time.

Aim to include a variety of rep ranges, with

- lower reps (one to eight) and heavier weights aimed at strength;

- higher reps (twelve to twenty-four) and lower weights or body weight aimed at size (more muscle, more benefits!);

- slow, explosive movements (such as plyometric exercises, including lateral hops, jump squats, and bounding) aimed at power.

I often use an interval timer and find a difficulty level where I can perform each exercise for one minute (about ten to twenty reps, for two to four sets). Speaking of difficulty, you can make your workouts progressively more challenging (to keep increasing your strength, endurance, and power) without any equipment at all by adding single-side exercises (like one-legged squats), plyometrics, or additional sets and reps.

Endurance Training

Whatever your aerobic activity of choice, such as biking, hiking, running, or swimming, a good metric to gauge your effort is the rate of perceived exertion (RPE) scale where

- 0 is lying in bed (minimal effort),
- 5 is walking briskly (moderate effort),
- 10 is running from a bear (maximum effort).

Again, try to include a variety of different endurance activities with varied intensities and lengths (like a leisurely forty-five-minute bike ride one day and fifteen minutes of hill sprints the next), with an emphasis on the lower end of the spectrum (an RPE of 3 to 5).

Mobility Training

When you regularly move your joints through their full range of motion, you have a greater capacity to safely engage with life's physical demands and opportunities. To build a body that's strong, expansive, and elastic, be sure to add mobility exercises to your resistance and endurance training programs — and include these three areas (in a two-, three-, or four-to-one ratio to posterior-chain stretches):

- Anterior-chain stretches (like a back extension or dancer's pose), which elongate your front

- Lateral plane stretches (like a seated side bend or exalted warrior), which elongate the sides of your body

- Transverse plane stretches (like a seated or supine twist), which improve your ability to twist

Now complete the exercise at the end of this chapter to create your own movement schedule!

SO THERE you have it: the multifaceted movement principles to weave throughout your day! When you combine the elements of physical activity, breath, posture, strength, endurance, and mobility, you will not only transform the health of your brain and body, but also expand your sense of personal power. And now that we've worked up an appetite, it's time to eat!

TENETS OF FEELING BETTER: MOVEMENT

- **Physical activity:** Start an anti-sedentary revolution by weaving movement throughout your day.

- **Breath:** Practice the 1-2-3 Breathing technique (always through your nose) to build energy, increase focus, and activate your parasympathetic nervous system.

- **Posture:** Take up more space. Your alignment affects the functioning of all body systems, as well as your sense of personal power.

- **Strength:** Build and maintain your skeletal muscles with a focus on posterior-chain and multi-muscle exercises.

- **Endurance:** Challenge your heart and lungs with a variety of cardiovascular exercises, especially walking.

- **Mobility:** Maintain the range of motion in your joints, with a focus on anterior-chain, lateral plane, and transverse plane movements.

Consider the 3 As

1. **Ask:** Which movements can you weave throughout your day? In your journal, write down the movement snacks, meals, and feasts you can schedule this week, then put them in your calendar.

2. **Affirm** the significance of movement. In your journal, write down three or more benefits you experienced from moving your body.

3. **Act:** Practice, and reflect on, movement rituals in a flexible framework. In your journal, write down the physical activities you did, then confirm how that made you feel.

CHAPTER 6

Nourish Your Body

*"Life is about fulfillment. If your life isn't fulfilled,
your stomach can never supply what's missing."*
DEEPAK CHOPRA

A FEW YEARS ago, I ran an online workshop called "The Art of Energy Management," which asked participants to take an audit of their overall energy levels, identify their energy zappers, and get clear on their energy boosters. One of the top energy zappers? Low-performance fuel. One of the top energy boosters? Nourishment.

To nourish is to provide yourself with the fuel necessary for wellbeing. Energy is the power derived from the use of that fuel. Low-performance fuel, such as highly processed foods, diminishes your energy. If you want to gain more energy from your nutrition, you need to consider the following:

1. **Menu:** what you take in
2. **Receptivity:** how you take it in
3. **Digestion:** how you process it

Because we can't quit eating, as we can quit other habits that deter us from achieving our dreams, we have to shift the way we think about food to help shift our behaviour. To act in your own best interests and grow your sense of power, you need high-performance fuel. This isn't a revolutionary idea — that we need to eat well to feel well (and perform well) — so what's holding us back?

I honestly can't think of a single person I know who hasn't struggled with this, or a working parent who isn't regularly stressed about mealtime and lacking the energy to make positive changes. In the post-workshop survey, 85 per cent of respondents said they were not happy with their overall energy. And answers to my question "What's holding you back from having more energy?" included the following. See if any resonate with you.

- "Not prioritizing myself and what fuels me and a lack of good meal prep."
- "Bad habits and emotional eating."
- "Not having a consistent schedule and poor time management."
- "I still eat sugar even though I know it doesn't work for my body."
- "So much stress in our family right now."

- "Lack of child care is holding me back."
- "Long workdays and too many demands on my time."
- "My own lack of action. I need to expend energy to get energy, but it can be hard to get started."
- "I have the knowledge but struggle in taking action."
- "Not sticking to a routine. I seem to constantly rebel against routine."
- "Lack of discipline and setting boundaries."
- "I don't always prioritize meal planning, so my energy is used up planning things on a daily basis."
- "Stress, anxiety, feeling overwhelmed with a long to-do list."

What *is* revolutionary is reprioritizing the rituals we have around nourishment, rethinking the kind of fuel we're putting into our bodies, questioning the marketing messages that enable bad habits, and making space to reflect on the outcomes of our choices. We need to rewild our nutrition.

Every day you are exposed to multiple messages that promise food should be fast. Flashy packaging grabs your attention and clever marketing grabs your cash. Hyperpalatable foods — also known as fast food, processed food, and junk food (i.e., low-performance fuel) — are manufactured in a lab to have an irresistible combination of sugar, fat, carbohydrates, and salt.

But these foods are never satiating, and good food is never that fast. We're forever unsatisfied when we consume low-performance fuel because it's designed to make us want more and more. It's energy-dense (high in calories) but nutrient-poor (lacking the building blocks our body needs), and temporarily lights up our reward centre like fireworks, before the harrowing crash into biochemical oblivion.

You must become mindful of the *aftermath* of consumption if you truly want to change your behaviour. To nourish yourself is more of a slow fix than a quick fix, but I'm here to help you make this process much speedier and more efficient — more indulgent and delicious.

"Really thinking about how food is fuel has been the biggest shift for me," said my long-time client Sarah, an angel investor and mom of a young child, who's been prioritizing the exercise of pausing, reflecting, and asking herself these two questions: "How am I feeling?" and "What has contributed to this good or bad feeling?" As she told me, "When I am on point with my nutrition, I have more energy for my workouts and life in general, I feel satisfied and not all-consumed by food, I feel happier, and I feel capable of making better choices. When I'm feeling off track with my nutrition, the first thing I do is start writing down what's going on. This self-accountability is key."

Even if you despise journaling and refuse to do it for any other part of this book, I implore you to give it a go for at least twenty-one days if you'd like to better nourish yourself. Doing this will make it clear how to remove the food-related barriers that are holding you back from having more vitality.

I struggled with binge eating in my teens and twenties, and nothing helped me shift my behaviour until I started taking notes on the reasons for and results of my unhealthy choices. It always felt excruciatingly hard as I embarked on a new "healthy diet" and was completely consumed with cravings, like an addict needing a fix. And then suddenly, I had no cravings and had gained wellsprings of willpower — all thanks to self-directed neuroplasticity (and my trusty journal).

This is why we have to take a combination Type 1/Type 2 Fun approach to food. Your taste buds will always choose hyperpalatable foods because, well, they're hyperpalatable! You must choose on your body's behalf and simultaneously hold space for discomfort and delight — both constructive pleasure and constructive pain. Look for the greatest variety of foods that taste good *and* are good for your biochemistry.

Food literacy is the knowledge to make informed choices and the skills to adequately nourish yourself. You must become exceptionally competent in nourishing yourself, which means recruiting both mind and body to the campaign. By tuning into how you feel mentally and physically after a meal, you can shift your cravings from low-performance fuel to high-performance fuel, and better understand what truly satiates you.

This is where we must begin, with our receptivity to nourishment.

RECEPTIVITY

The mindset and the history you have with food influences what you choose to eat. But the *way* you eat is just as important as what ends up on your plate. To satiate is to satisfy a need or desire. Food can fill the hole in your tummy, but it doesn't always fill the hole in your heart. When you approach meal planning, meal preparation, and meal consumption as an act of love and nurturance, you'll find you are more receptive to its offerings.

For this, you may have to do some reparenting. Perhaps your caregivers didn't have a healthy relationship with food. Either they ate poorly or they were too rigid so that eating has become fraught with all sorts of rules and behaviours that are affecting how you nourish yourself today. If you find yourself unmindfully practicing the habits modeled by your caregivers, let me reassure you that you can choose a new mindset and create new rituals for yourself.

If your nervous system is in a state of chronic sympathetic activation, this can affect how you digest and absorb your food, setting you up for all kinds of health issues. As I talked about in chapter 2, you need to feel safe and connected so that your nervous system can shift into parasympathetic activation. Prior to setting the table, you need to (mind)set the stage for physical and psychological safety, and for connection with yourself, with whomever you are eating, and the living things (plants and animals) you choose to ingest.

Mealtime Communion

To commune is to exchange intimacy and closeness. We have become so rushed and distracted that we've disconnected from this important part of nourishment. When you slow down at mealtime, you apply the parasympathetic brakes and engage the capacities of your digestive system for absorption, your metabolic system for utilization, and your nervous system for fellowship.

I am fortunate to have grown up with daily family meals around the dining table, cooked from scratch by my amazing mom. This was a nonnegotiable ritual I brought to my marriage, and now I am modelling this sense of unrushed closeness with my child in the way we savour food and prioritize presence around the table. I also like to involve my daughter in the meal planning and preparation, beginning with the adventure of discovering the raw ingredients available to us — an important part of any food literacy curriculum. We visit farmers' markets, subscribe to community-supported agriculture (CSA) boxes, peruse the produce section at the grocery store, and care for our family plot at the community garden.

"Young children are restless seekers who are satiated only when allowed to feast on human connection," says clinical counsellor Deborah MacNamara in one of my favourite parenting books, *Rest, Play, Grow*. This need for human connection is true for adults too. "Being attached," says MacNamara, "is the answer to our greatest hunger as human beings." To activate your body's rest-and-digest response so that you can satisfy your hunger for nourishment, you must first feel safe and connected.

I believe that the presence of digital devices at mealtime is diminishing our sense of safety and connection. The next time you're at a restaurant, take a tally of the families where every child and adult has their eyes locked onto a screen (and their hearts closed to each other). It's very sad indeed.

What's so bad about screen time during mealtime? It's much easier to disappear into your phone than to apply the energy needed for thoughtful conversation. And it's much easier to give the kids a tablet to keep them quiet and occupied, especially at dinnertime, when you're tired and have accrued big feelings from the various stresses you've endured throughout the day. However, there's a significant cost to this disconnection from ourselves and each other. Remember that every action influences your nervous system and is reinforcing patterns in your brain (same for those you're responsible to care for). Are you reinforcing

- **distraction or connection?** Not being present and engaged blocks you from human connection.

- **unmindfulness or mindfulness?** Eating without awareness blocks you from considering what you're taking in and how it makes you feel.

- **multitasking or uni-tasking?** Doing multiple things while you eat activates the fight-or-flight response and blocks the rest-and-digest response.

- **destructive pleasure or constructive pain?** Succumbing to the immediate reward of hyperpalatable foods blocks you from embracing the potential discomfort of healthier choices.

- **sympathetic activation or parasympathetic activation?** Not slowing down to savour the simple pleasure of a good meal blocks your receptivity to nourishment.

These are just a few of the reasons I've enacted a #diningroomdeviceban, and I invite you to join me! Everyone benefits from the intention to connect at mealtime — even if, at first, it feels like Type 2 Fun.

MENU

I want to assure you that I'm no culinary masochist, demanding you deprive yourself of deliciousness. I arrived at my first menu guideline after I left my full-time fitness job and began freelancing as a food, wine, and cocktail writer. This line of work was completely opposite to the land of bodybuilding, where boiled chicken and steamed broccoli reigned supreme. I have absolutely nothing against quality protein and cruciferous vegetables — far from it — but it was the fact that those "fitness diets" were defined by blandness, denial, and a lack of flexibility. I stepped back to look at the whole spectrum and saw that no one at either extreme was particularly happy or healthy. There had to be a thriving middle ground between stark deprivation and overindulgence. And that's when I started developing the following menu guidelines.

1. The Ratio Rule

As both a gastronome and a wellbeing enthusiast, I was determined to create a guiding principle that was sustainable for a lifetime and that banished the all-or-nothing mentality. The Ratio Rule, which takes into account nourishment of mind, body, and spirit, asks you to forget about removing anything "bad" and to focus on adding more "good." For example, I follow the 70/30 rule, where 70 per cent of meals are designed to fuel my mind and body with high-performance fuel and 30 per cent of meals allow for the addition of spirit fuel (including a little ice cream, cookies, chips, wine, beer, and whisky). How do you know if something is spirit fuel? Because it elevates, rather than dispirits, you.

My journaling practice has made eating a mindful ritual, one where I acknowledge that everything I put into my body is a choice. This process, which I'm continually refining, has allowed me to elevate my spirit fuel; I'm now very happy with one square of fair-trade dark chocolate instead of my old favourite, a king-size candy bar. I rarely overeat, thanks to reflecting on the destructive pleasures that lead to food comas and a bloated belly. And I've become very moderate with my indulgences — I'm deeply satisfied with one glass of wine.

Whether you're starting from 51/49 or 80/20, I'm excited for you to define your ratio and discover what fuels your mind, body, and spirit. The remaining menu guidelines will focus on mind-body fuel.

2. Meal Design

One of the keys to being *physically* satiated is to find your ideal balance of the three types of macronutrients: protein, fat, and carbohydrates. This takes some experimenting, but the return on investment is very high: a lifetime of more energy and vitality.

Protein is the cornerstone of satiety, so I start there. The recommended dietary allowance (RDA) for protein for sedentary adults is 0.8 grams per kilogram of body weight per day, whereas the American College of Sports Medicine's current recommendations for active adults (which I hope you've now become!) is 1.2 to 2.0 grams of protein per kilogram of body weight per day. For example, a person who weighs 65 kilograms (143 pounds) should aim for a minimum of 78 grams of protein per day, or 26 grams per meal (breakfast, lunch, and dinner). Your efforts to build more muscle by exercising more won't be realized unless you also consume adequate, good-quality protein.

To determine your ideal amount of protein per meal, use this formula:

[Your body weight (in kilograms) × 1.2 to 2.0 (you can experiment to determine what feels good to you)] / 3 (meals) = grams of protein per meal.

To determine amounts for the other macronutrients and sculpt a meal that sticks, start from the current acceptable macronutrient distribution ranges (AMDRs) for adults of 10 to 35 per cent protein, 45 to 65 per cent carbohydrates, and 20 to 35 per cent fat. Over time, I have arrived at a meal design of 35/45/20, which I've simplified to fractions of my plate: a little over a third for protein and a little under two-thirds for carbs, with a smidge of fat. Let me further explain my shortcut to omnivorous meal design.

Carbohydrates include starch, fibre, and simple sugars; proteins include animal-based and plant-based sources; and dietary fats include saturated fat and unsaturated fat. There is some overlap (especially if you're vegan), as some carbohydrates have protein, and some proteins have fat — and not all macronutrients are created equal.

The carbohydrates to focus on adding to your diet are

- fibrous vegetables,
- starchy vegetables,
- legumes,
- whole grains.

The fats to focus on adding are

- unsaturated fats, such as unrefined oil (cold-pressed olive, avocado, or canola);
- nuts;
- seeds.

If you are an omnivore, focus on adding proteins higher in unsaturated fats, such as grass-fed beef and dairy, pastured pigs who forage, free-range bison and chicken, and sustainable fatty fish and shellfish (that are also low in mercury) like salmon, trout, sardines, shrimp, clams, and oysters. What about micronutrients: vitamins and minerals? If you eat a variety of primarily local, organically grown foods in a rainbow of colours, you'll likely cover all of your micronutrient bases.

Here's what a weekday of three omnivorous meals containing about 26 grams of protein each could look like:

- **Breakfast** (650 calories): one piece of sourdough toast with peanut butter, a fried egg topped with an ounce of cheese and a big sprig of parsley, and a cup of kale salad with olive oil and sea salt

- **Lunch** (850 calories): three ounces of chicken with two-thirds of a cup of sourdough pasta, tossed with one cup of arugula, a quarter cup of chickpeas, a handful of halved cherry tomatoes, a pinch of rosemary leaves, a glug of good olive oil, and six chopped walnuts, plus a half cup of sautéed brussels sprouts

- **Dinner** (650 calories): three ounces of steak with a cup of sautéed broccoli and a cup of roasted sweet potato, topped with a tablespoon of pumpkin seeds

As you can deduce from my above sample daily menu, it provides about 2,150 nutrient-dense calories per day. You need to have sufficient daily calorie intake (especially when you switch from processed foods to whole foods and increase your physical activity) to feel fabulous instead of lethargic.

How long should a meal stick? Ideally at least four hours. Try experimenting with the ratio of macronutrients to find what satiates you. Blood sugar regulation is directly related to mood regulation — whacky blood sugar leads to whacky moods. If you're hungry an hour or two after you've eaten, you likely need to add more protein, fibre, and/or fat to your meal. How do you know what to add? You can discover your own unique nutritional needs through the trial and error of journaling!

3. Create Rituals

One of the keys to being *emotionally* satiated is to ask yourself what you're really hungry for. When you eat, you are nourishing more than your body. As I mentioned earlier, mealtime communion is such a worthy ritual to put in place, even if you begin with just one meal per week. It's an act of love to prepare, serve, or share a meal with those we cherish — even when dining alone, you are an important recipient of this love. This generous act takes time and intention. Often attributed to Benjamin Franklin is the adage "Failing to plan is planning to fail." In the words of my client Sarah: "Planning has helped me most in creating these positive shifts. When I purposely set myself up for success, it's hard to slip back into bad habits."

When we become overwhelmed with multiple responsibilities and the mental load of keeping every plate spinning, our nutrition is often the first thing to suffer. Meal planning is an efficient way to ensure we've done the upfront work to have everything we need available to nourish ourselves throughout the week.

Every Sunday, I map out each meal for the week ahead, make a grocery list from that plan, and place an online order to arrive on Monday, where I then organize my fridge, freezer, and pantry so that the ingredients are prepped and ready to go. If I don't do this, there's a high likelihood of me ordering a lot of pizza.

It's worth repeating that writing down how you feel after you eat can be the quickest fix to shift your habits — thank you, self-directed neuroplasticity! If you want to improve the way you eat, here's my invitation to you: for twenty-one days, for at least one meal per day, write down how you feel 30, 60, 90, 120, and 240 minutes after you eat — even if you just take mental notes. Journaling is a very powerful tool to help you design adequate meals to better nourish yourself and those you care for.

4. Investigate the Origins of Your Food

Before I started my freelance career writing about food for local and international media outlets, I trusted all those marketing gimmicks designed to make you feel good about what you were buying. "Free-run!" That must be good, right? "High fibre!" It must be healthy, right? But the veil was lifted when I investigated how things were really made. As my writing focused on sustainable agriculture and the ethical treatment of animals, I drove around to farms outside many of the cities I visited to see firsthand how things were done. When we talk about energy as the power derived from the fuel we eat, it's important to think about the energy we're incorporating into our being. Just watch a few undercover videos on gestation crates, or the sterile, unloving, and greedy production of hyperpalatable processed foods, and you'll never look at what you eat the same way again.

Just as it's our responsibility to provide movement opportunities for our children, it's our responsibility to be aware of the costs of our foods' production. There are so many simple and beautiful ways to connect with high-impact nutrition (better for you and the planet) and amplify the influence of mindfulness to nourish yourself better. In Western Canada, where I live, my preferred supplier is SPUD (Sustainable Produce Urban Delivery), because they deliver organically grown food to my door and rely heavily on local producers and in-season products. SPUD shows me both the vendor's bio and the kilometres travelled for each item so I know who I am buying from and supporting and can tally my carbon footprint for each grocery order.

5. Cut Out Junk

How do you know if it's junk? Ask yourself if the food resembles the form in which it was created by nature. For example, an apple versus those garbage fish crackers. The former comes straight from a tree; has edible packaging; has only one ingredient; and is a good source of fibre, vitamin C, and antioxidants. But the latter comes from a package that goes into the landfill and has twenty-one processed ingredients, none of which is high-performance fuel.

I could rant on and on about nutrient-poor, hyper-palatable kids' snacks marketed to make parents believe they're a reasonable choice, but I want to briefly step down from my soapbox to acknowledge that some of my spirit fuel comes in a package too. I guess that's my point: when you bring mindfulness to your choices, you become aware of exactly what you are putting into your mouth and the bodies of those you care for.

6. Circadian Fasting

Cleanses were so hot when I was in my teens and twenties, and I tried them all in the hopes of shedding weight and "detoxing" what was left of my body. I always felt sluggish, angry, and, inevitably, like a failure because they were impossible to stick with. In my thirties, when I'd shifted my focus to brain gains instead of weight loss, I kept hearing about caloric restriction and its link to longevity, so I began digging into the research.

At the time, I was still struggling with my sleep and with emotional eating, and intermittent fasting (going for periods of twelve to forty-eight hours without food) looked like a promising practice. But still, I couldn't get through an energetically demanding workday without eating and not feel terrible. That's when I discovered circadian fasting (also called time-restricted eating) and it perfectly aligned with my desire to extend my health span, improve my sleep, reduce my consumption of low-performance fuel (emotional eating generally happens at night), better balance my hormones, and boost my athletic performance.

Circadian fasting is simply extending the time between your last meal of the day and your first meal of the next day, and is an extension of circadian health — recognizing that all organ systems have a daily schedule and aligning our habits to best serve them. According to an article in the journal *Cell Metabolism*, "time-restricted eating is an emerging dietary intervention that aims to maintain a consistent daily cycle of feeding and fasting to support robust circadian rhythms. Circadian regulation of the endocrine system, autonomic nervous system, and nutrient metabolism contributes to metabolic and physiological homeostasis."

Here is how it works for me: Five days a week, I eat at 7:30 a.m., 12:00 p.m., and 4:30 p.m. — and never snack — leaving four and a half hours between each meal and allowing for a fifteen-hour overnight fast. Two days a week, I happily indulge in some evening snacks, and sometimes oblige my friends who like to eat dinner at 6:30 p.m.

If you choose to try circadian fasting, what length of time should you aim for? That depends on a number of factors, including your age, activity level, existing medical conditions, and the phase of your cycle (if you menstruate). Use your journal to track how you feel and speak to your doctor if you have any concerns. A very important point to note is that any type of fasting lifestyle must provide *adequate nutrition*. This is not about starving yourself; it's about nourishing yourself, giving your digestive system a break, and allowing your body's important overnight repair jobs to function optimally. Plus, it encourages you to question the kind of nourishment you truly need. Ice cream can never replace a hug, and a bag of chips can never replace feeling valued and validated.

7. Start a Love Affair with Your Kitchen (and Dishes)

If you're the one who's driving your family's nourishment train, you may be spending more time in your kitchen. To make your time there more pleasant, invest in nice things like fancy dish gloves and fabulous-smelling dish soap.

Take time to set up systems and stations so everything you need is readily available, and up the entertainment ante with people, music, or podcasts you love. You can also maximize efficiency by batch cooking. I make every meal in quadruplicate so it feeds our family two dinners and two lunches, which means I only have to cook every other night.

8. Avoid Food Waste
While I generally stick close to my weekly meal plan, I also practice what I call "refrigerator triage" — using up what's about to expire first. Good food is an investment, and it pains me to buy groceries only to throw them away. Apparently, I'm not the only one who's ended up tossing a neglected, slimy container of greens. According to the Food and Agriculture Organization of the United Nations, 14 per cent of the world's food — valued at $400 billion dollars — is lost annually between harvest and the retail market, and of the remaining food that makes it to market, 17 per cent is wasted at the retail and consumer level. These losses and their associated environmental, social, and economic impacts, reports the United Nations Environment Programme, are responsible for 10 per cent of global greenhouse gas emissions.

DIGESTION

My husband and I were together for eleven years before we got a dog, and for nineteen years before we had a kid. Until that point, we had never discussed bowel movements with each other. To be honest, I hadn't really thought a lot about it myself until I started toting around poo bags and changing diapers. Any time my dog or child had a suboptimal poop, I would retrace the previous twenty-four hours to try and figure out why. I started to do the same for myself and suggest the same for my clients.

It turns out that monitoring what you eliminate can be a great indicator of wellbeing. This is a good practice to start with your kids when they're young so you can normalize talking about bodily functions. I love the extremely teachable moment that November 1 brings each year — the day after Halloween and a few days after her birthday — when I explain to my daughter why her normally textbook-perfect poops look and smell so awful, thanks to the excessive consumption of hyperpalatable junk food, which differs from her normal diet.

All of these considerations got me thinking about how we can also look at nourishment beginning with the end in mind. Here are six tips for the best poops ever:

1 **Water:** Hydration affects more than just digestion and elimination. Studies have linked dehydration with reduced cognitive function, fatigue, depression, and anxiety. Do you remember the lawn waterslide that you had to soak with the garden hose? Think of your digestive system like that childhood favourite and don't forget to turn on the hose (by drinking adequate water) so that waste can easily slide right out of your body. How much water is enough? It depends on how much you talk, sing, snore, sweat, or mouth breathe,

and how much water content is in the food you eat. A great gauge is to look at the colour of your urine — it should be very pale and odourless. Darker and strong-smelling urine can be a sign of dehydration (which is normal first thing in the morning).

2. **Movement:** Physical activity stimulates peristalsis (the involuntary muscular contraction that moves food through your gastrointestinal tract) to help digestion, absorption, metabolism, and elimination — so don't forget to stay committed to the anti-sedentary revolution!

3. **Alignment:** Expansive posture is also important to the aforementioned bodily functions. If there are kinks in your internal hoses, thanks to compression and poor posture, this can lead to trouble delivering nourishment and exiting waste.

4. **Prebiotics:** Some of the fibrous foods we eat *feed* the helpful bacteria that make up our microbiome (the microorganisms that live in our gut). Examples include flaxseeds, seaweed, leafy greens, apples, almonds, bananas, oats, onions, and garlic.

5. **Probiotics:** Some of the foods we eat *add* helpful bacteria themselves to our microbiome. Examples include fermented foods (found in most traditional cultures) like kimchi, kombucha, miso, pickled vegetables, sauerkraut, tempeh, and yogurt, plus fresh (that is, local and in season), organically grown fruits and vegetables whose own microbiomes have remained largely intact.

6. **Parasympathetic activation:** Remember that the fight-or-flight response causes our body to power down the systems that aren't essential during a life-or-death situation (including the immune, reproductive, and digestive systems), so that energy can be rerouted to power up the musculoskeletal system and mobilize us to act. Your body will not prioritize digestion, absorption, metabolism, and elimination if you're distracted by sympathetic activation. Use the tools you've learned so far to engage the recovery response before you bring your fork to your mouth. Just taking a few deep breaths and saying a few words of gratitude can help shift you into a receptive mode. Take it to the next level when you slow down, remove distractions, gather together, and savour each bite.

In the next chapter, I will show you how to amplify the benefits of all these nourishment upgrades by getting adequate rest (remember parasympathetic activation is also known as the rest-and-digest response). You will learn how quality sleep can boost your metabolism, whereas poor sleep can undermine your quest to eat better through disruption of your appetite hormones, setting you on a path of unchecked hunger and excess energy intake.

TENETS OF FEELING BETTER: NOURISHMENT

- Increase your receptivity to nourishment with the tools you have for parasympathetic activation, such as mindful breathing, mealtime communion, and a #diningroomdeviceban.

- Invest in creating a weekly meal plan to save time and money, and maximize your nutrition.

- Focus on adding more high-performance fuel to your plate.

- Include protein, prebiotics (fibrous foods), probiotics (especially local, in-season, organically grown fruits and vegetables), and unsaturated fats.

- Use your journal to discover your ideal ratio of macronutrients and length of circadian fasting.

Consider the 3 As

1. **Ask:** What kind of nourishment can you add throughout your day? In your journal, write down the menu plan and grocery list for this week; then order what you need, and put the meals in your calendar.

2. **Affirm** the significance of nourishing yourself. In your journal, write down three or more benefits you experienced from nourishing your body.

3. **Act:** Practice, and reflect on, nourishment rituals in a flexible framework. In your journal, write down the nourishment rituals you practiced, then confirm how that made you feel.

CHAPTER 7

Rest Your Body

*"Rest is radical because it disrupts the
lie that we are not doing enough."*
TRICIA HERSEY

"I FEEL ABSOLUTELY terrible in so many ways when I am sleep deprived," said my client Brooke, a podcaster, author, and mom to three teenagers. "When I am overtired, everything is an issue, every problem feels insurmountable. I don't feel like I can get through the day, I don't want to exercise or eat properly, and tasks take way longer to complete than they should."

How many of us have similar struggles? Nearly everyone I talk to is tired. It is wild to rest and recharge!

Just as exercise is only part of movement, and what you eat is only part of nourishment, sleep is only part of rest. When you rest, you activate your parasympathetic nervous system's recovery response, allowing your body to achieve homeostasis: the state of balance between body systems required for optimal functioning. Without adequate rest, your body must work much harder and expend more energy to maintain homeostasis. Inadequate rest, especially sleep deprivation, breaks us down emotionally, cognitively, and physically.

Fatigue can impair your capacity for learning, memory, attention, problem-solving, decision-making, mental flexibility, and self-control, as well as your capacity for kindness, compassion, and presence in the relationships you have with yourself and others. "I do not do well with sleep deprivation," said my client Julia, who has two young children and is finishing her master's degree in clinical counselling. "I am a bad version of myself. I have a hard time concentrating, finishing my schoolwork, and being patient with the people in my life. I tend to drink more coffee (which makes me anxious and irritated), skip my workouts, drive instead of walk to pick up my kids from school, and make poor meal choices. I am harder on myself when I haven't slept and get extra emotional over little things."

Sleep deprivation also has a wide range of physical costs, including hormone imbalances that negatively affect appetite, metabolism, and fertility; detrimental changes to gut microbiota; impaired workout recovery; reduced pain tolerance; and decreased immune function. In this chapter, I want to show you how small shifts to your sleep hygiene and intentional rest practices can build up your physical, emotional, and cognitive wellbeing.

THE PRO-RECOVERY REVOLUTION

Intentional rest is your commitment to daily recovery practices that provide opportunities for you to relax, repair, renew, restore, and reinvigorate. But not all rest is horizontal! Intentional rest can be active or passive, solitary or social. Here's what I mean by that:

- **Social active rest:** This is moderate-to-high-energy activities with other people, such as playing pickleball, attending a group fitness class, going on a family hike or group cycling ride, or lively sexy time with a special person.

- **Solitary active rest:** This is moderate-to-high-energy activities but done solo, such as running, gardening, practicing yoga, or lifting weights.

- **Social passive rest:** This is low-energy activities spent in company, such as sharing a meal, watching a movie, playing board games, cuddling with your people, or having coffee with a friend.

- **Solitary passive rest:** This is low-energy activities done solo, such as reading, doing puzzles, colouring, having a bath, savouring a cup of tea, listening to the rain, watching the sun rise, or, of course, sleeping.

"Intentional rest has become an essential component of my life since I came to your retreat," Julia told me. "My meditation practice has improved significantly. Some days, it's two minutes; other days, it's twenty minutes. I listen to my mind and body and go from there. I like to spend time by myself each day with a coffee on my living room couch. I don't use my phone. I grab a magazine or my Kindle and set a timer for thirty minutes to enjoy my coffee and read uninterrupted. Another important shift has been quality time with my kids and husband. My phone has been going on do-not-disturb at dinnertime, and I don't touch it until 8:00 a.m. the following morning. Our mealtimes are now uninterrupted, *and* they are true family time: we have beautiful conversations together around the table. Plus, sexy time with my husband has improved *tenfold*."

To protect your commitment to the pro-recovery revolution, you need strong boundaries like Julia created. To diagnose if you are suffering from inadequate rest, examine the inner and outer barriers in the way of your recovery, and the inner and outer boundaries you have in place to pave the way to recovery.

I had the pleasure of hearing author Elizabeth Gilbert speak about her book *Big Magic*. She said that an aha moment came to her with the realization that from the long list of words we hear to describe women — Strong! Badass! Fierce! Vulnerable! Wholehearted! — the one that's never included is "relaxed."

But it's important we understand how to achieve a state of relaxation more regularly, because we can't be fully present, access our well of wisdom, and operate from a place of compassion and creativity without parasympathetic nervous system activation. "The most powerful person in the room," said Gilbert, "is the most relaxed person in the room." In other words, your ability to effect change can be diminished when you're depleted. It's necessary — and not selfish — to prioritize rest in order to truly make positive change in your own life, and in the world.

To do this, said Gilbert, you need to put three things in place: figure out your priorities, protect them with boundaries, and connect with your intuition (or another massively loving and knowing force you believe in) through some kind of contemplative practice, like meditation or journaling, for guidance on how to take action.

This is exactly what my client Brooke did. "For many years, I have felt the benefits of taking time to rest, either by having a fifteen-minute nap, meditating, listening to music, or letting myself sleep until I know I am rested." She added, "My whole family knows that when I say I need a nap, I need it, and they honour that. But it took a while for them to respect that boundary."

When you prioritize rest, you not only become a more relaxed and powerful version of yourself, but also catapult your creativity to another level.

DELIBERATE REST STIMULATES AND SUSTAINS CREATIVITY

Maybe you've heard of the 10,000-hour rule (achieving expertise in a particular skill by practicing for at least ten thousand hours). But there's a lot more to this pop-culture soundbite, says Silicon Valley–based consultant Alex Soojung-Kim Pang, author of *Rest*. World-class performance, he says, "comes after 10,000 hours of deliberate practice, 12,500 hours of deliberate rest, and 30,000 hours of sleep."

Allowing your mind to temporarily shift focus away from the task you're tackling, and having had a good sleep, can help you crystalize the swirl of ideas in your head. In fact, says Pang, "mind-wandering is the secret of creativity" and an important part of creative breakthroughs, which follow a four-stage process:

1 **Preparation:** gathering information

2 **Incubation:** subconsciously considering that information while focused on other things

3 **Illumination:** the aha moment when you arrive at the answer

4 **Verification:** confirming and polishing the new creative concept

"Whether they know it or not," says Pang, "creative people treat incubation and illumination like skills every day. That's why they develop and refine daily routines and practices that preserve time for mind-wandering, sharpen their sensitivity to insights, and allow them to capture moments of illumination."

Now, how do you get those thirty thousand hours of sleep? You develop and refine daily practices that allow you to wind down so you can fall asleep, stay asleep, and wake up feeling refreshed.

NEW FRONTIERS IN SLEEP SCIENCE

Sleep hygiene is an important part of overall hygiene, which is defined by the World Health Organization as practices that help maintain health and prevent the spread of disease. If you've ever let sleep hygiene slide down your priority list, you should know about your *glymphatic system* — and no, I didn't spell that incorrectly!

A massive leap in our understanding of why sleep is so important to wellbeing and longevity came in 2012, when a team of researchers led by neuroscientist Maiken Nedergaard discovered what's now known as the glymphatic system. Our body's lymphatic system, a vital part of our immune system that serves to remove metabolic waste, pathogens, and cancerous cells, doesn't extend to our brain. Instead, non-neuronal cells in the central nervous system, called glial cells, take on this role. "Intriguingly," the researchers noted, "the glymphatic system functions mainly during sleep and is largely disengaged during wakefulness."

In chapter 5, I told you how although the brain comprises only 2 per cent of your body weight, it consumes up to 25 per cent of the energy that you take in. And what does energy consumption produce? Waste. And in our brain, lots of it. In his TED Talk, Nedergaard's colleague, neuroscientist Jeffrey Iliff, says that during sleep the glymphatic system "shifts into a kind of cleaning mode to clear away the waste from the spaces between its cells, the waste that's accumulated throughout the day." Without this nightly custodial work, the brain becomes clogged, foggy, less focused and productive, and at greater risk for neurodegenerative diseases like Alzheimer's and Parkinson's.

Structural changes associated with neurodegeneration can begin to occur twenty-five years before the first symptoms appear or a clinical diagnosis is possible, so it's important to do everything in your power *today* to engage your glymphatic system — and every other regenerative system in your body — through consistent, quality sleep. Quality sleep also boosts the "fountain of youth" I mentioned in chapter 5: growth hormone.

The quality of your sleep is also a major determinant of all of the choices you make in a day, from the moment you wake up:

- whether or not to exercise
- the quality of your nutrition
- the amount of water you drink
- how physically active you are throughout the day
- how creative and focused you are
- how kind and compassionate you are
- how present and patient you are
- how you'll approach bedtime — and set the stage for the next day

What does quality sleep look like? For adults, the guidelines are seven to nine hours per night. How do you know where you fall along that spectrum? Go to bed at the same time for a few nights in a row, don't set an alarm, and note what time you wake up naturally.

I know that my body requires seven hours of sleep, and that if I honour my sleep hygiene practices (more on that below), it takes me less than thirty minutes to fall asleep. With a lights-out time of 9:30 p.m., I reliably wake up around 5:00 a.m., which gives me about ninety minutes for my morning rituals before my daughter wakes up around 6:30 a.m.

Turning out the lights at the same time every night might feel like a challenge if your current schedule isn't marked by regularity, but this may be the most important sleep hygiene factor to consider, for you and your family. And if you are curious about how much sleep your children might need, here are the recommendations over a twenty-four-hour period, including nighttime sleep and daytime naps:

- Infants (4–12 months old): 12–16 hours
- Toddlers (1–2 years old): 11–14 hours
- Children (3–5 years old): 10–13 hours
- Children (6–12 years old): 9–12 hours
- Teenagers (13–18 years old): 8–10 hours

A 2024 paper in the journal *Sleep* reports that even when "adjusted for age, sex, ethnicity, and sociodemographic, lifestyle, and health factors... sleep regularity was a stronger predictor of all-cause mortality than sleep duration." The authors also stated that "people with irregular sleep patterns are exposed to irregular patterns of environmental stimuli, including light, and may have irregularly timed behaviours, such as physical activity and meals. This unstable timing of both stimuli and behaviours leads to disruption of circadian rhythms, with downstream negative health effects," say the authors.

Your body has a master clock — located in a small part of the brain called the *hypothalamus* — that regulates your daily cycles, also known as your *circadian rhythm*. This master clock modulates the individual biological clocks for every one of your organ systems, and relies on both internal (physical activity, diet, stress) and external (light and dark) stimuli to regulate itself. Every morning, especially if you slept poorly, ate or drank late, and/or were exposed to unnatural light after sunset, you can help resynchronize your clock with exposure to sunlight — one more reason an outdoor walk in the morning is one of the best things you can do for your wellbeing.

I touched on the idea of circadian health in chapter 6, and I believe it's hugely important in rewilding yourself. If you're feeling overwhelmed about reclaiming your wellbeing, focus on restoring your circadian rhythm first. This approach to health means aligning your habits — in a regular, cyclical pattern — with the light-dark cycle of the time zone you're in, to allow all of your body systems to function and repair within their own optimal schedules. Abiding by circadian health can be boiled down to a very simple directive: move and eat within an eight-to-twelve-hour window when it's light outside, and rest when it's dark.

An ideal daily schedule by which to set your protective boundaries might look like exposing yourself to natural light early in the morning, moving your body here and there throughout the day, eating within a window of less than twelve hours, and winding down to give yourself the best chance of getting seven to nine hours of sleep.

In his book on unleashing the power of circadian health practices, Satchin Panda, a professor at the Salk Institute for Biological Studies, says:

> It is hard enough for the body to monitor hormones, genes, and clocks for someone with a strict eating routine. But when eating occurs at random times throughout the day and night, the fat-making process stays on all the time. At the same time, glucose created from digested carbohydrates floods our blood and the liver becomes inefficient in its ability to absorb glucose. If this continues for a few days, blood glucose continues to rise and reaches the danger zone of prediabetes or diabetes. So, if you've wondered why diets haven't worked for you before, timing might be the reason. Even if you were diligently exercising; counting calories; avoiding fats, carbs, and sweets; and piling on the protein, it's quite likely that you weren't respecting your circadian clocks. If you eat late at night or start breakfast at a wildly different time each morning, you are constantly throwing your body out of sync. Don't worry, the fix is equally simple: Just set an eating routine and stick to it. Timing is everything.

Now, I'm not telling you to disregard all of the wonderful nourishment information that I shared in the last chapter, but to make a point on the importance of timing, I want to share an interesting element from Panda's TED Talk, "Circadian Code to Extend Longevity." His lab studied a group of overweight adults who chose a ten-hour eating window that worked for their lifestyle each day, during which they ate everything they wanted for a period of sixteen weeks. They not only lost a significant amount of weight and maintained that weight loss a year later, but also reported that they were sleeping better, had less joint pain — which made them feel better *and* allowed them to exercise more — and felt more energetic throughout the day.

The incredible domino effect of aligning my habits with my circadian rhythm is the reason I have only JOMO, never FOMO, when I retreat to the quiet, dimly lit, unplugged sanctuary of my home at 4:30 p.m. for dinnertime most nights.

SLEEP HYGIENE FOR THE WIN!

Sleep hygiene practices allow you to wind down at night and rev up in the morning to better support your circadian health, wellbeing, and longevity.

Here are nine sleep hygiene practices (divided into three categories) you can choose to experiment with to give yourself the best chance of having a fantastic sleep. I say the *best chance* because many factors are often out of our control. As I write this chapter, I am struggling with sleep loss because my fifteen-year-old dog is struggling with a long list of health problems, including snoring loudly (in my bed), and vomiting or falling down the stairs in the middle of the night. And to any sleep-deprived parents with a newborn baby or toddler — or anyone else with sleep disruptions that are out of your control — remember that all these practices fall along a spectrum that can expand or contract based on the current moment. This is about doing everything in your power to have the best *quality* sleep possible, even when the *quantity* may be less than ideal.

First, let's set the stage by having a look around the room where you sleep.

Sanctuary

Without spending too much time or money, it's possible to transform your bedroom so that it instills a mindset shift when you walk through the door: *This is a sacred space for rest.* Here are the three things to consider when you're upgrading your space.

1. **Cool:** Body temperature naturally dips when we sleep, and a room that's too hot can make it harder for our body to make this important shift. Providing a cool environment can include turning the heat down, cracking a window open, sleeping naked, and/or investing in bedding with natural fibres that breathe.

2. **Calm:** Unleash your inner interior designer and go for a luxe spa hotel vibe, with relaxing colours, textures, lighting, and scents, and uncluttered décor, plus blackout curtains (I'll explain why in a moment).

3. **Purposeful:** A bustling multi-purpose room for working, exercising, watching movies, and storing junk is not the vibe you are going for in your sacred space for rest. As you cross the threshold into the bedroom,

leave your worries behind and relax into a space that's designed for peaceful activities like reading, meditating, journaling, orgasms, and, of course, sleep.

Now consider the kinds of rituals you create to help you wind down at night and rev up in the morning.

Evening Rituals

Intentional rest practices can help keep your cortisol at manageable levels so that when it comes time to sleep, you don't have an insurmountable mountain of that stress hormone circulating in your body. Cortisol has an inverse relationship with the sleep hormone melatonin, meaning one must be low for the other to be effective. You can facilitate this natural daily seesaw by inspecting the varied sources of stress in your life, and individually tweaking them to reduce your overall stress load. Here are three ways to do that.

1 **Disconnect:** Thanks to mobile devices, many of us are available to incoming messages from multiple sources 24-7. But you can choose to disconnect from the people, devices, conversations, and worries that keep your sympathetic nervous system activated. You can put the brakes on and engage your parasympathetic nervous system by giving yourself the auditory, visual, mental, emotional, and cognitive rest you need.

"A good night's sleep is a total game-changer," said my client Yvonne, who previously struggled to disconnect from the day's stresses in the evening. "I love having PM rituals and don't know how I managed so long without them!"

she said. "Unplugging from digital devices at the end and start of my day is an intentional rest practice I've been working on, and I've included my son in creating these rituals to ensure we understand each other's goals. We agreed on a solution that works for both of us and it has made all the difference. I've noticed a change in my mental, physical, and emotional health when I do unplug."

2. **Wind down:** Once you've addressed the outside sources of stress, turn inward to further wind down. As mentioned in the last chapter, aim to reduce your nutritional stress by eating dinner earlier — with your last bite or sip ideally a few hours before your head hits the pillow. Try downloading (writing down) anything that's adding to your mental load. Years ago, my husband and I developed a team guideline to shelve hard conversations after 7:30 p.m. and revisit them earlier the next day. We found that hashing out a disagreement late at night was generally never worth the sleep loss this invigorating activity usually led to.

3. **Dark:** Light is the strongest external stimuli to your master clock. Your eyes have millions of light detectors, and so does your skin. When light is sensed, melatonin is suppressed, signalling to your body that it's not time to sleep — even though you might be trying to convince it otherwise by putting your head on your pillow. Modern humans spend an average of 90 per cent of our time indoors and, thanks to electricity, we can be exposed to unnatural light for much of that time, which is one of the largest contributors to circadian dysregulation. Often, after the

sun sets — when our ancestors would have used fire and candlelight, followed by absolute darkness — our evening activities include screens that emit blue light, the most stimulating form of light on the spectrum (whereas red light is the least stimulating) and keep our cortisol high. To counteract the negative effects, if you must look at screens in the evening, try dimming them as much as possible and changing the display to a warmer colour; and try swapping alarm clocks and night lights with blue lights to those with red lights. When it's finally time to sleep, equip your bedroom with blackout blinds so outside lights can't interfere with your sleep quality.

Morning Rituals

Your day's choices are largely impacted by the quality of sleep you've had, so it's wise to spend at least a minute upon waking analyzing your sleep quality and quantity and reverse engineering why it may have been good or bad — to inform your choices for the day and night ahead. Brooke said, "If I've slept well, it's easy for me to get up and not hit the snooze button. I then do my morning rituals, including gratitude journaling, meditation, deep breathing, and drinking water, followed by a cup of coffee and breakfast. When I get my AM rituals done, I feel like the rest of my day has the potential to be productive and enjoyable. If I feel tired or rushed and can't take this time for myself, I feel way more anxious." Here are some ideas for creating your own morning rituals.

1. **Connect:** After you wake, before you plug back into society, take some time to connect with yourself. What kind of sleep did you have? How are your energy levels? What are your intentions for the day? What's most important to you? What are you grateful for? What's the big-picture vision you have for your life, and what small steps can you take today to move in that direction? In other words, just as you may choose not to consume food for the last few hours of the day, you can choose not to consume media for the first few hours of the day. If that suggestion made your knuckles turn white, remember we're operating in the flexible framework — start from wherever you find yourself right now (even just five minutes).

2. **Rev up:** After you connect with your mind and spirit, this is a great time to connect with your body. Stretch it, strengthen it, move it in any way that feels good. I love to follow a workout with a hot shower finished with an invigorating cold blast and indulge in a quick head-to-toe moisturizing skincare routine. Then I love to fuel myself with a big, hearty breakfast and savour my first meal of the day with my family, preferably outside on the covered patio, even if that means wearing our parkas in the winter.

3. **Light:** Exposing myself to natural light early in the morning is only one of the reasons I love to dine alfresco, but it's a really good reason. If your lifestyle is contributing to circadian dysregulation, one of the

simplest things you can do to press the reset button and regain circadian health is get outside in the morning, whether that includes having a stretch on your patio, having breakfast in the open air, or going for a walk. Even if it's cloudy, being outdoors can help resynchronize your master clock. And if you're feeling groggy, early morning exposure to light is a quick way to lower your melatonin, allowing cortisol to help you feel more alert.

REST IS more than just activating your parasympathetic nervous system. To rest is a spiritual practice that goes beyond the emotional, physical, and cognitive realms. Rest is an act of liberation that connects us with our true essence, our humanity, and our sovereignty. Says the "nap bishop," Tricia Hersey, author of *Rest Is Resistance*, "Our liberation is deeply connected to the portal of healing we can tap into when we rest. There is synergy, interconnectedness, and deep communal healing within our rest movement. We will not be able to interrupt the machine of grind culture alone. We need each other in more ways than we are allowed to believe. This work is about radical community care."

In the next chapter, we will continue to explore the power of connection, communal healing, and radical community care.

TENETS OF FEELING BETTER: REST

- The pro-recovery revolution includes intentional rest practices that are active or passive, solitary or social.
- Deliberate rest stimulates and sustains creativity.
- Your glymphatic system works during sleep to clean out your brain, and this is critical to reducing your risk for neurodegenerative diseases.
- Sleep regularity is key to circadian health, but if you get off track you can help resynchronize your clock with exposure to morning sunlight.
- Sleep hygiene practices include creating a sanctuary for sleep, evening rituals that help you wind down, and morning rituals that help you rev up.

Consider the 3 As

1. **Ask:** What kind of rest can you add throughout your day? In your journal, write down the active, passive, social, and solitary rest you can schedule in your calendar this week.
2. **Affirm** the significance of rest. In your journal, write down three or more benefits you experienced from being well-rested.
3. **Act:** Practice, and reflect on, rest rituals in a flexible framework. In your journal, write down the rest rituals you practiced, then confirm how that made you feel.

CHAPTER 8

Connect with Other Bodies

"For once we begin to feel deeply all the aspects of our lives, we begin to demand from ourselves and from our life-pursuits that they feel in accordance with that joy which we know ourselves to be capable of."
AUDRE LORDE

I SAT TALL in my chair, craning my neck to get a better view of the famous physician speaking onstage before a large audience at a love-and-relationship summit in Vancouver. He and his wife of fifty-five years were delivering the conference keynote, titled "Reconciling Attachment with Authenticity." Gabor Maté and Rae Maté were both generous and pragmatic in sharing their not-without-challenges life and relationship arc, and the universality of a "traumatic tension" that affects each and every one of us: our concurrent need for both attachment and authenticity. It was refreshing and comforting to know that at the age of eighty, this bestselling author and global expert on stress, addiction, trauma, and childhood development was still reconciling this inner struggle.

In his book *The Myth of Normal*, Maté says that attachment is our instinct to secure both physical and emotional proximity to others, and to facilitate caretaking. This instinct is shaped in childhood but carries through to all parts of our adult life. Our earliest attachment relationships can impact both our personal and professional lives, often unconsciously, and not always to our benefit. If you had to sacrifice your authenticity to secure attachment as a child, you may continue to unconsciously do the same as an adult if you don't question the truth of who you really are.

To be authentic is to be wild, to be aligned with your true nature, to embrace the full expression of your whole being. As you continue the process of rewilding, you are becoming your authentic self. Rewilding your social connections requires rooting in that integrity of self while consciously growing strong branches of attachment in your diverse ecosystem of relationships, ranging from partnership and parenting to community and connection with nature.

Let me begin with parenting, as the relationship between parent and child serves as both an act of tremendous generosity to our offspring and an exercise in curiosity that — with mindfulness and grace — can alert us to our own wounds of inauthenticity.

REPARENTING TO REBUILD ATTACHMENT AND AUTHENTICITY

Whether you have children or not, you have a beautiful opportunity to reparent yourself and create the ideal environment for self-healing and self-actualization. In any relationship, you can keep the concurrent need for both attachment and authenticity top of mind, as you navigate how to model self-regulation, boundary-setting, and self-leadership.

This is what my client Mia, an event planner and mom to a preteen, is learning to do. "I am starting to grow in the area of authenticity, and my husband isn't. He is stuck in the mindset that he's supposed to be a certain way because his parents told him this, and his grandparents told him this, and the world wants him to be in this little box. It's very difficult for the two of us, especially as parents," she told me through tears.

"I see it in the way we talk to our son, and I can't believe we've treated a child like that. I'm afraid to let my son be who he wants to be because of my own fears, and my husband is afraid he won't fit into the mould that is expected. I don't want my son to be in that place when he is in high school or an adult. My husband and I both need to be more conscious of this, but we have to do it together, as a family."

I, too, struggle with this balance in my own parenting. It's not an easy path to hold space and remain calm in the face of big feelings and conflicting ideas. It's not an easy path to emancipate yourself from cultural and familial programming. It's not an easy path to uphold the boundaries you've created to maintain wellbeing for everyone in your household when you're tired, depleted, and overwhelmed. But consciously creating an environment where both authenticity and attachment can thrive is the path to breaking free from negative patterns, and perhaps ending cycles of intergenerational trauma that kept your ancestors from aligning with their own authenticity — and from experiencing the joy of deep attachment. You can lead the repair crew that liberates your lineage.

"Repair is one of my favourite words in parenting," says clinical psychologist Becky Kennedy, author of *Good Inside*. "There's no such thing as a perfect parent," she says of the moments where we fall short, the moments we regret. "Our parenting doesn't have to be defined by our moments of struggle; it should be defined by whether or not we connect with our kids after the struggle, and whether we explore how those moments felt to them and work to repair the rupture in the relationship."

When you repair — and this goes for adult relationships too — you are rewiring the experience of the conflict with a sense of safety and understanding. The key element of repair, says Dr. Becky (as she's known on social media), is *connection after disconnection*. "When we return to a moment that felt bad and add connection and emotional safety, we actually change the memory in the body. This limits your child's tendency to self-blame and sets [them] up for a stronger relationship with you and also healthier adult relationships."

You can offer this experience of repair to yourself too. In your journal, or with someone you trust, you can return to a moment that felt bad and reframe it, allowing yourself to release self-criticism and reinforce self-healing.

RECRUITING YOUR SUPPORTING CAST

None of us can live a good life alone. Even our household units can't thrive in isolation. It truly takes a village to raise a family. As I mentioned in chapter 2, we moved a lot during my childhood and were without extended family or established community. My dad worked full time, and my mom stayed at home, single-handedly managing every aspect of our domestic, school, and extracurricular life, with nary a complaint. This no doubt took a toll on her wellbeing.

I both complained and raged after having my daughter, as I deeply felt just how much weight the mental load is for many women to bear — especially as the cost of living soars past the average income, necessitating for most families that everyone secures a source of income, essentially doubling a family's workload. Yes, things are shifting, and I'm fortunate to have a partner who is shedding the layers of cultural programming alongside me, but even with greater equity within the home, it's too heavy for a family unit to bear alone. We must consciously build our own villages of support.

"Every parent needs a supporting cast, and the less one exists naturally, the more it needs to be cultivated by design," says psychologist Gordon Neufeld in the book he co-authored with Maté, *Hold On to Your Kids*.

"Many adults now in their forties or beyond recall childhoods in which the village of attachments was a reality," he says of the neighbours, friends, and extended family who acted as surrogate parents. But for many of us today, "that attachment village no longer exists."

Every human needs a supporting cast, and you must cultivate this by design. You must diversify and deepen your relationship ecosystem, while staying true to your authentic nature. "The stress of self-suppression may disturb our physiology, including the immune system," says Maté. Self-expression, on the other hand, can delight your physiology — especially when received by a strong supporting cast.

The suppression of negative emotions like anger, jealousy, fear, and frustration is a stressor that's detrimental to our physiological and psychological wellbeing, and so is the suppression of positive emotions like joy, gratitude, pride, and awe. "I have this inner battle of wanting to be true to the ridiculous and playful authentic me, while being afraid of not being accepted, afraid of talking too much, afraid of saying the wrong thing," said my client Angela, a communications specialist. She continued:

> I often feel like I don't fit in. I am the most ridiculous person at the government organization I work for, which is pretty corporate and stoic. They don't quite know what to do with me. But if I can't work somewhere where I can actually be truly me most of the time, then it's not going to feel good. I've just made that conscious decision to be authentic and true to myself. That

being said, I have a new boss who doesn't "know" me yet, and it has triggered my people-pleasing and wanting-to-fit-in tendencies, so I'm working through that.

Whether you feel like you don't fit in at work or don't stack up to everyone else on social media, you can still feel alone even when your connections are many.

THE STRESS BUFFER OF RELATIONSHIPS

In 2023, US Surgeon General Vivek Murthy released an advisory on the public health crisis of loneliness, isolation, and lack of connection. "Given the significant health consequences of loneliness and isolation," said Murthy, "we must prioritize building social connection the same way we have prioritized other critical public health issues such as tobacco, obesity, and substance use disorders. ... Our relationships are a source of healing and wellbeing hiding in plain sight — one that can help us live healthier, more fulfilled, and more productive lives."

Loneliness — being physically or emotionally isolated from each other and/or feeling detached from our authentic selves — fuels multiple billion-dollar industries as people consume drugs, junk food, media, home décor, fast fashion, and electronic gadgets to try and fill the holes in their hearts. But what truly fills those holes is positive relationships. And a meta-analysis on social support and longevity suggests that relationships have a stress-buffering effect on us. Positive relationships can not only reduce our risk of mental disorders and physical disease but also increase our lifespan.

The opposite of social isolation is *social integration*. Social integration, as I shared with you in chapter 4, encompasses a large spectrum in your relationship ecosystem. It includes small gestures like waving to your neighbour, making eye contact with the cashier at your grocery store, and conversing with other parents at school pickup, as well as larger gestures such as the lively discussions at your monthly book club, chit-chat with your co-workers in the lunchroom, and intimate conversations around the family table. The stress-buffering effects of social integration, say the researchers, include three neurobiological pathways:

- the autonomic nervous system (promoting parasympathetic dominance)
- the neuroendocrine system (dampening the effects of cortisol and boosting oxytocin)
- the immune system (decreasing proinflammatory proteins)

Interestingly, that stress buffer is strongest between parent and child during infancy and childhood, switches to friends during adolescence, and is "followed by a new and powerful romantic partner buffering effect in adulthood."

The power of social integration is great news. Even if you've just moved to a new city and feel like a stranger, or your social circle has fragmented and is restructuring, or if you feel socially isolated, you can always take action to boost your social integration and build community.

COMMUNITY: PLACE, PURPOSE, PEDIGREE, AND PROFESSION

A sense of community is a feeling of friendliness with other people who share commonalities. You can build community with your neighbours (place), fellow enthusiasts of particular passions (purpose), your family (pedigree), and your colleagues or clients (profession). To flourish, this and all parts of your relationship ecosystem need the loving attention of an expert gardener.

Connection rituals serve to nourish these relationships and attend to any care they may need. Whether you consider your community members friends or friendly acquaintances, your part in the quality of relationship you have with others, your ability to offer attention and care, and your capacity to be a calm and compassionate presence comes down to self-leadership — your awareness of and commitment to your own wellbeing.

One of the corporate workshops I offer is called "The 5 Cs of Great Leadership: How to Be Calm, Confident, Collaborative, Compassionate, and Creative." In this workshop, I explain nervous system regulation from the perspective of strengthening social bonds, using the somatic and cognitive tools that you've learned so far, including physical activity, rest, nourishment, breath, eye contact, posture, tone of voice, presence, active listening, laughing, singing, and physical affection (where appropriate).

Embodying each of the Cs requires you have the awareness, intention, and tools to flip into parasympathetic activation. But this ability to flip into parasympathetic activation isn't just applicable to your community relationships — it's also a crucial part of your intimate and personal relationships.

ROMANCE IS A VERB

I believe that romance is an action word — a verb, not a noun. Just like movement rituals are habits practiced to improve and maintain your strength, endurance, and flexibility, romance rituals are habits practiced to improve and maintain your love, desire, and intimacy with a partner.

I've long been interested in the rituals that keep romantic partnerships strong *and* spicy over time, not only in my work with coaching clients and my freelance writing career — I used to write love stories for a wedding magazine — but also in my own relationship. My husband and I had our first "date" when we were twelve years old. We went to see a movie with a group of friends but sat in the theatre holding hands like we were the only ones there.

We were separated at the end of that school year because of family moves, but miraculously we were reunited four years later when our families unexpectedly ended up in the same town again. My parents and I were visiting the local high schools to decide where I would attend Grade 12, and as we walked through the main doors of the last school, a voice over the intercom requested that my former crush please come to the office! I hadn't heard his name in years, and I rushed down the hallway to see if it was really him — it was. We've been together nearly every day since (approximately ten thousand of them).

MORE THAN a writer, coach, or speaker, I identify as a researcher. I love to learn everything I can — compiling, organizing, and linking data — about the things that interest me, and I am very interested in love. One of the most impactful books I read early on in my marriage was *Mating in Captivity* by Esther Perel. "Love seeks closeness, but desire needs distance," she says.

This polarity echoes Gabor Maté's thoughts on attachment versus authenticity. "Our need for togetherness exists alongside our need for separateness," says Perel.

> One does not exist without the other. The dual (and often conflicting) needs for connection and independence are a central theme in our developmental histories. Throughout childhood we struggle to find a delicate balance between our profound dependence on our primary caregivers and our need to carve out a sense of independence. We come to our adult relationships with an emotional memory box ready to be activated. The extent to which our childhood relationships nurture or obstruct both sets of needs will determine the vulnerabilities that we bring into our adult relationships — what we most want and what we most fear.

Many long-time couples develop unmindful patterns, where they aren't giving their full attention to connection or independence — leading them to feel unfulfilled in both areas. One of the most significant rituals my husband and I have adopted to prioritize our needs for both togetherness and separateness is to create a weekly schedule of personal nights and date nights. This way, our sense of self has space to flourish and our partnership has plenty of fuel to thrive.

You can grow the love and desire in your relationship by infusing every day with more aliveness and energy — what Sigmund Freud called *eros* and Perel calls *eroticism*. "Eroticism is a life force," says Perel, "an energy that infuses us with a sense of aliveness, of vibrancy, of vitality, of creativity, spontaneity, curiosity, imagination, and so much more."

Curiosity and excitement are essential elements to include in your romance rituals. To nurture the energy of eroticism in our life we must inject both the mundane and the extraordinary with simple pleasures and sensual delights that arouse our sight, hearing, taste, touch, and smell. Try incorporating more

- lightheartedness and play, like participating in games night or going dancing;
- culinary exploration, like cooking together or dining at a new restaurant;
- heart-pounding nature and athletic adventures, like snorkelling or beach volleyball;
- music and the arts, like going to a music festival or art gallery;

- physical affection and sexual activity, like giving a massage or trying a new sex toy.

A good recipe for a strong and spicy relationship that continues to support your own personal growth includes these energizing team pursuits, the honouring of individual differences, and a commitment to repair the inevitable ruptures that occur throughout life. And as with our human relationships, Dr. Becky's key element of repair — "connection after disconnection" — can, and I think must, be applied to our collective relationship with nature.

ENVIRONMENTAL STEWARDSHIP AS A SPIRITUAL PRACTICE

Stewardship is taking responsibility for and care of something. Just as we've learned to care for our own bodies in the last few chapters, we must also care for the body that we all rely on: Mother Earth. I believe so many of the world's problems are a direct result of disconnection from our humanity and a lack of daily practices that connect us with kindness and compassion to ourselves, to each other, and to the planet.

I define a spiritual practice as an intentional activity — a ritual — that deepens your relationship with your authentic self, connects you with universal oneness, and expands your capacity for love. Many of the rituals you've already learned to feel better in your body also serve as environmental stewardship practices. Here's a sustainable efficiency we should all abide by: what's good for people is generally good for the planet. Here are some examples:

- **Active transportation** — whether you walk or bike — increases your fitness while reducing your carbon footprint. Plus, morning exposure to sunlight helps sync your circadian clock, improves hormone regulation and immune function, and even prevents childhood myopia.

- **Green exercise** (a.k.a. nature workouts), as mentioned in chapter 5, multiplies the benefits of movement thanks to nature's impact on circadian health, immune function, stress management, and mental health.

- **Unstructured outdoor play** is one of the best things you can provide for your kids' psychological and physical development. It requires little planning on your part, doesn't use fossil fuels, and doesn't send junk to the landfill.

- Committing to the **anti-sedentary revolution** by doing yardwork and housework with your own two hands (like using a rake over a leaf-blower and hanging the laundry to dry instead of using the dryer) adds to your wellbeing and further reduces your carbon footprint.

- **High-impact nutrition** is better for you and the planet. Investigating the origin of your food inspires you to shop better and eat better, thereby reducing your environmental impact.

- Using **natural landscaping** by planting your garden with local flora — especially edible varieties — reduces water consumption and supports important species like bees. And as you become a co-creator of your diet, you also improve your gut microbiome. If you don't have a yard, try container gardening (herbs are a great place to start) or sign up for a plot at your local community garden.

- When you connect with your authenticity, express gratitude for what you have, and take the time to sit with difficult emotions, you help reduce feelings that may lead to **unconscious consumption** and **unchecked consumerism.**

- Embracing underconsumption and purchasing **sustainably made or used** clothing and home décor can improve air quality, divert waste from the landfill, and support fair wages and working conditions for the people who labour to create them.

- Reducing the use of **electronics and artificial light** decreases your use of natural resources, sends less waste to the landfill, increases your sleep quality, and lowers your stress load.

Imagine if we all made just a few of these shifts to our lifestyles! These sustainable practices have the power to move us toward the harmonious coexistence of human life and Earth's biosphere (the sum of all ecosystems). This harmony is described in the definition of "biophilia": humans' innate attraction to nature, our attachment to and love for living things. Rewilding is a return to this true nature, the recognition of oneness, the restoration of connectedness.

CONNECT WITH BODIES OF WATER AND LAND

As journalist Chelsey Luger and photographer Thosh Collins, wellness advocates and authors of *The Seven Circles*, say:

> Remember that at one time, in everyone's history, our ancestors were intimately connected to the land. The beautiful and unique aspects of every culture on earth resulted from our interacting with the beautiful, diverse natural regions from where we came. For many, that connection has been severed, and this continues to impact collective health and wellness today. It is imperative that we repair these bonds. [The land] is a life-giver, guardian, the root of all creation, the heart of the universe, and the essence of our very being. When she suffers, so do we. The health of the land is a direct reflection of the health of the people.

You can repair these bonds and reinstate an intimate connection to the land in so many of the rituals you practice each day, month, and season. Luger and Collins suggest engaging with the land by beginning "to observe seasonal changes and inherent characteristics of your environment, including animal behaviour, plant behaviour, weather patterns, sunrise and sunset, moon cycles, solstice, and equinox."

Try connecting with the elements of fire, water, earth, and air by taking inspiration from cultural practices that revere nature around the world, such as Indigenous sweat lodges in the Americas, Scandinavian wood-fired saunas, natural hot springs like Iceland's Blue Lagoon, and the Japanese practice of *shinrin-yoku*, otherwise known as "forest bathing" or taking in the natural surroundings with all your senses. You can enhance your connection to nature through the sensuality of immersive experiences like pressing your bare feet into the dirt, deeply inhaling the salty ocean air, staring into the crackling flames of a campfire, dining outside with the breeze against your skin, gazing up at the stars on a dark night, floating on top of a quiet lake, dunking yourself in an icy river, or listening to the cacophony of bugs and birds in an alpine meadow.

"Every day, our relationship with nature, or the lack of it, influences our lives," says journalist Richard Louv in *The Nature Principle*. "This has always been true. But in the twenty-first century, our survival, or 'thrival,' will require a transformative framework for that relationship, a reunion of humans with the rest of nature."

AS I will discuss in the next chapter, our "thrival" is an urgent matter that affects not only the quality and quantity of our own precious life, but also the legacy we leave for those who will call us ancestors.

TENETS OF FEELING BETTER: CONNECTION

- You can reparent yourself to rebuild authenticity and attachment.

- Every relationship can benefit from the intentional ritual of connection after disconnection.

- Recruiting your supporting cast, increasing the quality of your stress-buffering relationships, and reducing the harmful effects of loneliness take intention and presence.

- Intimacy in all your relationships, including in your romantic partnership, requires self-leadership, especially the commitment to your own wellbeing so that you can embody the 5 Cs of great leadership.

- Consider environmental stewardship as a spiritual practice to deepen your connection with nature.

Consider the 3 As

1. **Ask:** What connection rituals can you add throughout your day? In your journal, write down the family, community, and romantic rituals you can schedule in your calendar this week.

2. **Affirm** the significance of connection. In your journal, write down three or more benefits you experienced from being well-connected.

3. **Act:** Practice, and reflect on, connection rituals in a flexible framework. In your journal, write down the connection rituals you practiced, then confirm how that made you feel.

REVERENCE

A deep respect for someone or something

CHAPTER 9

Zoom Out: Lovingkindness, Longevity, and Legacy

"If our children are to approve of themselves, they must see that we approve of ourselves."
MAYA ANGELOU

"WE ONLY have this one life, and I know if I don't make these changes now, I'm going to look back and regret it," said my client Claire, an entrepreneur and mother of two young children. "What this experience has taught me is that life is so short, but there's so much we can do to have this rich, beautiful, juicy life — and it takes work like everything else. But if you put in the work, the beauty that can come from that is going to be magnified by a thousand. And I want that. I don't want a minute of my life to go wasted. I want to do the most I can do with this short time on Earth."

How rich, beautiful, and juicy could your life get? Close your eyes and imagine what it feels like to live as your truest self. Vibrant, happy, fulfilled. Love is the solution to this reunion with the true you! Do you love yourself enough to really do this — to invest in this quest and experience how good it can get?

Lovingkindness is a practice of directing good wishes to ourselves and others, of holding reverence for the preciousness of life, of accepting that we matter just because we exist. It's a trait that you can strengthen inside yourself to fuel forward motion.

Earlier in the book, I explained how what you focus on shapes your brain (chapter 3). Meditation is the practice of training your attention, of expanding the quality of your awareness, of maintaining a point of focus. Lovingkindness meditation is the practice of focusing on a few phrases that state what you most wish for yourself, such as "May I be safe, may I be happy, may I be healthy." This practice can help transform your inner dialogue, which can often be a roadblock to living the life you desire.

Everyone has an inner critic and an inner cheerleader. Our inner critic — also known as self-doubt, self-criticism, and self-sabotage — is the voice of fear. Our inner cheerleader — also known as self-trust, self-forgiveness, and self-leadership — is the voice of love. There is only love or fear. Notice which energy you're operating from and choose to pass the microphone from your inner critic to your inner cheerleader.

Lovingkindness meditation is one of the practices I used to flip the script on my nasty inner narrative and respond to my mistakes with the gentleness and grace I'd give my own sweet child or best friend. It's really powerful when you notice that there's suddenly a positive voice cheering you on inside your head. You can do this for yourself in just a few minutes of practice per day.

You are now equipped with more than a dozen cognitive and somatic tools to transform your mental and physical wellbeing, and an understanding of how to shift from knowing to doing. But it's critically important that you move through this new season of your life with extraordinary tenderness, radical acceptance, and tremendous courage.

The bridge from knowing to doing is paved with the following:

- **Mindfulness:** the awareness of what's constructive versus destructive and the recognition of reality, such as what's working and what's not working

- **Compassion:** the desire to alleviate suffering; curiosity and care without judgement

- **Strength:** the capacity to withstand difficulty and discomfort and the power to resist harmful forces

In order to construct a sturdy bridge so that you can consistently enjoy an elevated level of wellbeing, it's sometimes necessary to zoom out and view your life as a loving observer. When you catch yourself feeling overwhelmed, depleted, or caught in a downward spiral, try using this mantra:

"Stop!
ZOOM OUT."

———————

From this vantage point, you can see the big picture:

- What really matters?
- What do you need to see?
- What action can you take right now?

From this vantage point, you can look back, with radical acceptance for your whole self: the child you were, the adult you are, the mistakes you've made, and the milestones you've achieved. Use the growth mindset to solidify the wisdom you've gained and to transform any guilt you may be holding on to. What have you learned? What tools do you have now to do things differently?

When you stop to zoom out, you can be present, with extraordinary tenderness for the challenges you're facing and the dreams you're working toward. One of the best tools to develop your attention, awareness, focus — your presence — is meditation. I've already introduced two types of meditation: lovingkindness meditation and my 1-2-3 Breathing technique (in chapter 5). Now I'd like to offer you a few more of my favourites.

First, I'd like to share the most helpful meditation tip I've ever learned. This tip comes from Buddhist meditation teacher Sharon Salzberg, author of *Real Happiness*. When I first tried to meditate in my late teens, I thought the purpose was to clear your mind, which I couldn't do, so I felt like a failure and stopped. After finishing my neuroscience degree, I learned about contemplative neuroscience (the study of meditation's potent effects on the mind, brain, and body), and I was encouraged to give it a go again based on the exciting research on presence, peace, and vitality I had read about.

BREATH VS. NOT BREATH

A clear mind isn't the purpose of meditation; it's a *focused* mind you're striving for. "The moment you realize you've been distracted is the magic moment," says Salzberg. "It's a chance to be really different, to try a new response — rather than tell yourself you're weak or undisciplined, or give up in frustration, simply let go and begin again. The act of beginning again is the essential art of the meditation practice. If you have to let go of distractions and begin again thousands of times, fine. That's not a roadblock to the practice — that *is* the practice. That's life: starting over, one breath at a time."

For any meditation, no matter the point of focus, there's the *thing* you're attending to, and everything else is *not-the-thing* (any thoughts, sensations, or sounds). During a breathing meditation, for example, says Salzberg, "When a thought arises that's strong enough to take your attention away from the breath, simply note it as *not breath*." This concept was incredibly liberating and helped me become a consistent meditator. Let's look at it in practice.

Bubble Up Meditation

This one I made up and is a precursor to the other types of meditation. As a mother, wife, pet parent, entrepreneur, and homeowner, I have a lot on my mind — as I'm sure you do too — and when I sit down to meditate, the pause often brings up important things I've forgotten. So

I always have a pen and paper nearby and allow myself the first few minutes of my meditation to write down whatever bubbles up before I get serious about focusing my attention.

Lovingkindness Meditation
Sit in a comfortable place where you are safe and undisturbed. Gently close your eyes and settle into a rhythm of unforced, expansive breathing. Picture your own beautiful smiling face with your mind's eye and slowly repeat a series of kind and loving wishes that are meaningful to you, such as "May I feel peace, may I feel joy, may I feel love." When you become distracted, have gratitude for this magic moment of awareness, and return to the wishes again and again.

1-2-3 Breathing Meditation
Sit in a comfortable place where you are safe and undisturbed. Gently close your eyes, and as you inhale, expand wide, deep, and tall, and as you exhale, contract your pelvic floor, waist, and ribs (flip back to chapter 5 if you'd like to review the details). After five to ten breaths, or when you are feeling comfortable with the breathing practice, begin to simply repeat the words "in" as you inhale and "out" as you exhale. When you become distracted, simply label the distraction as "not breath," let it go, and return to the breath — in and out.

Moving Meditation
If sitting still feels overwhelmingly hard, or you haven't moved your body enough today, choose a physical

activity with slow repetitive movements that you can do safely, such as swimming laps, walking, rowing, cycling, or practicing yoga, and where you can focus on something like your breath or a particular muscle or sensation. When you become distracted, quickly congratulate yourself for being mindful, and return to your point of focus.

ALL TYPES of meditation can create presence as you sharpen your focus, peace as you deactivate the fight-or-flight response, and vitality as you activate the recovery response. The practice of meditation can also nurture the quality of courage, says Buddhist nun Pema Chödrön, author of *How to Meditate*. "Over time," she says, "you will find yourself developing the courage to experience your emotional discomfort" and learn "how to get out of your own way long enough for there to be room for your own wisdom to manifest. Meditation helps us to clearly see ourselves and the habitual patterns that limit our life."

MEET YOUR WISER SELF

When you stop to zoom out, you can also look forward, with tremendous courage to step into the beautiful vision for your life.

It can feel defeating when it seems like you're revisiting the same challenges, but please take heart in knowing that with each subsequent pass, you've become stronger, wiser, and better equipped. This journey is an upward spiral, not a hamster wheel. Imagine what decades of being true to yourself might look like. Your *wiser self* is someone who's ascended the spiral and crossed the bridge, and can help pull you upward and forward. Your wiser self is your number one fan, someone who loves you unconditionally and wholeheartedly, someone who's been doing the work — consistently, determinedly, courageously — and can not only preview what it feels like to be there but also show you exactly how to arrive. Your wiser self is the future version of you who is committed to taking daily action in service of your wellbeing, and is living wholly, truly, and unabashedly in alignment with your basic needs and wildest dreams. You can use your imagination to converse with this version of yourself, allowing you to change your perspective and find insight you weren't aware you possessed.

"Cultivating the Wiser Self," created by psychotherapist Linda Graham, author of *Resilience*, is one of the most powerful visualization exercises I've ever done. It was introduced to me by my business coach and is paraphrased below.

Your wiser self is "a reliable inner resource of wisdom and resilience," says Graham, someone who can answer any question you bring to them, anytime you need help, guidance, or support. "As with any use of imagination to create inner resources," she says, "whatever you can imagine is real to the brain. The more you practice encountering your wiser self, the more reliably you will be able to evoke [their] wisdom as you respond to the challenges and difficulties of your life."

To evoke your wiser self:

- Sit in a comfortable place where you are safe and undisturbed.

- Gently close your eyes and settle into a rhythm of unforced, expansive breathing.

- Picture yourself standing on a beach, looking out at the ocean. Ground your feet in the sand and breathe deeply. In the distance you see a small island where your wiser self is waiting for you.

- Picture yourself floating across the water to meet them there.

Your wiser self greets you warmly. Notice how they look, their vibrancy and vitality, how they move. Your wiser self invites you to walk or sit with them. Take this time to ask them whatever questions come to mind that could help you walk their path. These could include the following:

- What do I need to know to bridge the gap between present-me and future-me (you, my wiser self)?

- How can I overcome a specific challenge I'm struggling with now?

- What can I do to better prioritize my wellbeing on a daily basis?

- What else do you want me to know?

When it's time to say goodbye to your wiser self, thank them for this experience and bid them farewell. Slowly, imagine floating back to the beach you started on. Feel the sand beneath your feet and breathe deeply. Gently open your eyes and take a moment to write down what you experienced.

The practice of encountering your wiser self can be a regular part of step 5 of the Magic Formula (chapter 4). Pause to reflect, revise, and recalibrate as you move toward that future vision of yourself.

This and all visualization practices have been shown to physically change the brain — activating the same neurons as the real experience — and provide what psychiatrist Norman Doidge, author of *The Brain's Healing Way*, calls *internal neurostimulation*. "Neurostimulation is effective in preparing the brain to build new circuits," he says. In other words, visualization practices can spark neuroplasticity and help you change your brain — and life — for the better.

SELF-LEADERSHIP: THE PATH TO LONGEVITY

Self-leadership is the process of leading yourself across the bridge, of staying committed to your own wellbeing, and paving the road to longevity.

Blue Zones are places in the world where people live exceptionally long lives. When researchers looked at the lifestyle factors that contributed to their longevity, they discovered that these concentrations of centenarians (people who are one hundred years old or older) exist in cultures that have remained wild. Their community values and the environment they live in support their fundamental needs for connection, nourishment, movement, and rest. "The bigger idea of Blue Zones," says journalist, author, and host of Netflix's *Live to 100: Secrets of the Blue Zones* Dan Buettner (who coined the term), "is don't try to change your behaviour, change your environment. That will last."

Lasting change for yourself and those you care about starts with you. If the company you keep, and the environment you live in, are not conducive to wellbeing and longevity, you will have an uphill battle. But simple shifts to your home and habits (like setting up your environment, as mentioned in chapter 5) can have a large and lasting impact.

I have seen this first-hand, with the oldest residents at the retirement home where I worked as the social and fitness director in my early twenties when I was newly married. One couple, in particular, I will never forget. Aged 98 and 102 years old, they had been together for decades, but they still walked around holding hands and let everyone know when they were going back to their room to "smooch." They were physically active throughout the day (going for walks, playing 8-ball pool, and attending my morning fitness classes), had a strong social circle, and knew how to relax (they attended all the entertainment activities I organized). I'm so grateful for the influence they unknowingly had on me, as I've since held the image of myself at 102, enjoying happy hour with my friends and smooching my husband.

When you have reverence for your life and wellbeing — and create space for connection, nourishment, movement, and rest — you may be unknowingly inspiring those around you to do the same. When you normalize physical activity, celebrate rest, and ritualize mealtime, you are creating an environment that supports longevity. You can be the source of rewilding in your family and community. This is a legacy worth leaving.

YOUR LEGACY AS AN INFLUENCER

Whether it's one little kid looking up to you or millions of people following you, you are an influencer. What you do influences others, and how you make them feel has an impact. By breaking destructive patterns, building healthy habits, replacing limiting thoughts with empowering beliefs, increasing your energy and vitality, resting when you need to, and learning how to regulate yourself so you can better access your kindness, compassion, and presence, you are not only helping yourself feel better, but also elevating everyone in your sphere of influence.

As you create this bigger, better, truer life for yourself, you are changing the legacy you leave behind. "The way I approach self-care is so much different since the retreat," said my client Eva, a content creator, wife, and mother of two young children. "I have been eating more colourful food, drinking more water, moving my body more, and taking time to celebrate me. I can feel it, and my family feels it too — my husband has noticed a big shift in how I am every day. I am more patient and present when I am with my kids."

As you learn to find a better balance in your life, you are creating a shortcut for those you love, a road map for them to follow. Eva said, "One of my biggest takeaways was to get outside and move my body. Not only have I been feeling better physically, but also my mental health has been so much better since I incorporated this daily movement ritual. This also comes with such a sense of pride too. I am so proud of myself for sticking to it!"

As you continue this journey, you will understand more and more that your quest is universal, and your dedication to the path will be a beacon for your wellness crew to locate you. "Taking time to connect with myself and with other people, of all walks of life, was so healing in its own way," Eva said. "We were all gathered at the retreat, and while we are all facing different struggles in life, and different journeys, we were all connected with the same goal: health and happiness. It was truly beautiful to see."

Now it's time to get really clear on what the future of your journey looks like. Let's zoom in to create your personal action plan — your micro-manifesto!

TENETS OF FEELING BETTER: LEGACY

- Do you love yourself enough to fully invest in this journey of rewilding?

- Learn to flip the script on your inner narrative (cheerleader vs. critic) and become more mindful, compassionate, and strong through the practice of meditation.

- When you catch yourself feeling caught in a downward spiral, use the mantra "Stop! ZOOM OUT" so that you can identify what really matters and what action you can take right now.

- Self-leadership is crossing the bridge from knowing to doing, staying committed to your wellbeing, consulting your wiser self, and paving the road to longevity.

- You can craft your legacy by breaking destructive patterns, building healthy habits, replacing limiting thoughts with empowering beliefs, increasing your energy and vitality, resting when you need to, and learning how to regulate yourself so you can better access your kindness, compassion, and presence.

Consider the 3 As

1. **Ask:** What rituals can you add to zoom out every day? In your journal, write down the lovingkindness, longevity, and legacy rituals you can schedule in your calendar this week.

2. **Affirm** the significance of reverence for your life. In your journal, write down three or more benefits you experienced from zooming out.

3. **Act:** Practice, and reflect on, lovingkindness, longevity, and legacy rituals in a flexible framework. In your journal, write down the rituals you practiced, then confirm how that made you feel.

CHAPTER 10

Zoom In: Your Personal Action Plan

"If we care about ourselves and don't want to suffer, we'll naturally be motivated to achieve our dreams and let go of behaviours that don't serve us anymore."

KRISTIN NEFF

YOU'RE HERE, you made it this far! You're wilder and more liberated, better regulated. You've met your wiser self and have seen a glimpse of the incredible adventure that lies ahead for you. You're shifting from knowing to doing, and now it's time to refine your toolkit so that you can write your wellness prescription, your action plan, the detailed road map to your dreams: your micro-manifesto.

I am so proud of you. I know this work takes courage, strength, and discipline. I believe in you with all my heart and am so grateful that, by investing in your own well-being, you are part of the change that's transforming the earth's collective energy from fear to love. Know that you are never alone: there is a vast community just like you, on their own journey to feeling better.

In addition to zooming out, part of this journey requires zooming in and getting specific, looking at your life through a microscope. Tiny details matter.

YOUR MICRO-MANIFESTO

The following is the final exercise that we do together at my multi-day wellness retreats and in my online coaching programs. Do not skip this step. This is your micro-manifesto.

A manifesto is more than an action plan: it's a prescriptive declaration of your dedication to the revolution; a written statement outlining your guiding principles; an expression of your commitment to liberation and legacy.

A micro-manifesto is

- simple yet specific,
- scheduled yet flexible,
- so small it can't help being sustainable.

Your micro-manifesto will look different from everyone else's because it is unique to you. Sometimes people leave with a few specific actions, like my non-negotiable rituals I shared with you earlier: move, meditate, and reflect every day (for five to sixty minutes) to feel happy, hopeful, and strong. Remember, a ritual is a deeply sincere set of habits practiced according to a prescribed order.

Sometimes people leave with a word that signifies a number of actions, like one woman in my coaching program who laminated a set of matching notecards that simply said "solitude" to place in her wallet, on her desk, in her kitchen, and next to her toothbrush. For her, solitude was something she craved but wasn't getting enough of in her life. Seeing that word throughout her day was a cue to make time for reading, meditating, exercising, and spending time in nature.

Whichever approach you take, don't forget to keep your coaching hat on.

YOU ARE A GREAT COACH

A great coach is someone who supports your growth and champions your dreams by asking good questions that

- illuminate your goals, barriers, and boundaries;
- encourage efficiency and accountability;
- provide big-picture counsel.

The Magic Formula is a self-coaching model to help you sustain momentum through constructive questioning, guided reflection, and data collection. You can use the following questions as thought exercises, or you can increase their potency — using the power of strategic repetition — by making them journal exercises as an action-plan precursor to better help you prepare your micro-manifesto. Look back and see the Magic Formula unfolding throughout the four sections of this book:

The Rescue: Discover — Build Awareness
- What do you truly want?
- What do you need to feel safe and connected?
- Which habits do you want to build or break?
- How can you use the seven mindset shifts to think — then act — differently?

The Revolution: Diagnose — Identify Issues
- What barriers have you identified and rectified?
- What boundaries have you created and stated?

The Rituals: Prescribe — Create a Plan, and Practice — Take Action
- How do your rituals fit into the flexible framework? Can they expand or contract? Do they have a Plan A, B, and C, and are they scheduled in your calendar?
- What is your personal mantra to help fuel action?
- How can you use curiosity when you feel your commitment waning?

**Reverence: Pause — Examine Results
and Re-examine Objectives**

- What made you feel good — or what would make you feel good in its aftermath?

- Double-check your definitions: Are you roused — instead of repelled — by discomfort (i.e., constructive pain)? What could you reframe as Type 2 Fun?

- How are you using mindfulness practices, such as meditation and journaling, to improve inner noticing (i.e., metacognition)?

- How often are you making time for data analysis, future visioning, and re-examining your objectives?

CREATING YOUR ACTION PLAN

Flip back through the book to take stock of what resonated most. Then, take another pass with a lens for pattern recognition and follow these steps:

1 What commonalities do you see? What trends do you notice?

2 Combine similar themes.

3 Make a list of the ideas that struck a chord, the somatic and cognitive tools that felt most significant to you, the practices that resonated the most.

4 Next, whittle your list down to a maximum of three guiding words or rituals.

5. Simplify your list to its smallest iteration, so it's exemplary of the flexible framework.

6. In your journal, write down your three words or rituals, followed by as much detail as possible in terms of when and where you will practice (your Plans A, B, and C), how long you will practice (your flexible framework), and how you will feel once you've taken action.

7. Add these words or rituals to your daily calendar.

Your list (your action plan, wellness prescription) should feel wild, liberating, doable, and delicious. This is your micro-manifesto!

EASY RESETS FOR GETTING BACK ON TRACK

Just like with the practice of meditation, the question isn't if you'll get off track, it's when. Noticing you're off-track is a magic moment. It's an opportunity to choose to return to your path, the path of wellbeing. Here are some exercises to help you recalibrate.

Coach Yourself

Ask yourself a series of constructive questions to inspire action. Perhaps you'll flip back through the book and pick a few of your favourites or create some of your own — so they're handy when you need a boost. The exercise at the end of chapter 4 is a great place to start: What do I know?

(Discover); What do I need? (Diagnose); What do I do? (Prescribe); How will I practice? (Practice); How did that feel? (Pause).

Consult Your Wiser Self

Review the instructions in chapter 9 to engage your wiser self, and ask them questions like "How can I get back on track?"; "What advice do you have for me today?"; or "How shall I proceed given the current circumstances?"

Visit Your Deathbed

I had a sobering moment last year when I realized our Dream Book had more pages left than we have years, even if we join the centenarian club. It made the present moment feel more urgent and provided the *activation energy* — the force that moves us from inaction to action — I needed to make better choices.

"Death is the most powerful reminder that there are only so many moments in a human life," say the authors of *The Tools*, psychiatrist Phil Stutz and psychotherapist Barry Michels. The fifth and final tool they share is called "jeopardy" and involves imagining your elderly self on your deathbed suddenly sitting up and screaming at you "not to waste the present moment," which makes you "feel a deep, hidden fear that you've been squandering your life."

This reminder is important to revisit regularly. Life is so precious, so finite, and your potential is limitless. "Your future is in jeopardy every moment," say the authors. "That generates tremendous urgency — and the willpower that comes with it. Willpower is the missing link in reaching human potential."

Build Community

As you continue moving forward, be sure to seek kindred spirits to join you on this journey. They may include your family, friends, and colleagues, or you may find camaraderie in an online community. I invite you to visit my website (thelifedelicious.ca) to register for freebies, online programs, and in-person events where you'll find kinship, inspiration, and accountability. And I hope you'll join my wildly successful and engaged community of alumni! Please share your *Feel Better Now* journey and find each other with the hashtag #FBNmicromanifesto.

TENETS OF FEELING BETTER: ACTION PLAN

- Celebrate the steps you've already taken to become wilder, more liberated, and better regulated.
- Know that you are never alone: you are part of a vast community of amazing humans, just like you, on their own journey to feeling better.
- Your micro-manifesto is a prescriptive declaration of your dedication to the revolution; a written statement outlining your guiding principles; an expression of your commitment to liberation and legacy.
- Does your micro-manifesto feel wild, liberating, doable, and delicious?
- You can always rely on the great coach you have inside yourself!

Consider the 3 As

1. **Ask:** What rituals make up your micro-manifesto? In your journal, write down your new rituals in as much detail as possible.
2. **Affirm** the significance of practicing them. In your journal, write down three or more benefits of practicing these rituals.
3. **Act:** Practice, and reflect on, the power of these daily actions to help you feel better. In your journal, write down the rituals you practiced, then confirm how that made you feel.

Conclusion

"Do whatever brings you to life."
ELIZABETH GILBERT

YOU ARE now equipped with the tools to become unstoppable. Each new moment, and every new breath, offers the opportunity to choose forward motion, to fuel the upward spiral, to remain unstuck. Consistency no longer eludes you.

You have the power — every minute of every day — to reassess the quality of your life, and recalibrate accordingly. Rewilding is a radical approach to *rescuing* yourself from the systems that keep you unwell, unmindful, and unsatisfied. And your liberation from suffering supports collective liberation.

Your regulation supports co-regulation. Your boundaries inspire those around you to create their own. Your self-leadership allows you to show up as the most calm, confident, collaborative, compassionate, and creative version of yourself, transforming all your relationships. Your reparenting serves as a model to others.

This liberation, this *transformation*, arises when you can

- recognize patterns of unmindfulness vs. mindfulness;
- shift from knowing to doing, from consumer to creator of your life;
- facilitate self-directed neuroplasticity vs. experience-dependent neuroplasticity to hardwire healthy habits;
- become aware of simple, flexible, everyday opportunities to complete the stress cycle, promoting rest and recovery.

Rewilding is the return to your true nature, the celebration of your authenticity. It is the practice of caring for all parts of yourself, using the tools I've shared with you in these pages.

Your authentic self is truly a thing of beauty. And so is the integrity of self in those you're surrounded by. Consciously creating the community, environment, and rituals to support collective wellbeing is an urgent matter. You are now part of the *revolution* that favours a new system — a more simple, satisfying, and indulgent way of living, a legacy of slowing down and savouring the abundance around you.

This journey is not without hardship. It's especially important that you identify the invisible barriers that threaten to derail you, such as limiting beliefs, self-criticism, discomfort, mild adversity, busyness, and fear. Nothing exonerates you from facing challenges; we all must surmount the inevitable stresses of life. But you are strong enough to persist. And when your sturdiness is challenged, or when you get off-track, you can turn to the inner and outer resources you always have available to you. These include the following:

- your micro-manifesto, with detailed instructions for daily wellbeing

- your journal, with empirical evidence confirming what serves you and what doesn't

- your commitment to, and discipline of, awareness, reflection, and lifelong learning, so you can rouse inspiration inside yourself

- your connection with your wiser self, the future version of you who has taken daily action in service of your wellbeing, who has already navigated and overcome the challenges you are facing, who has already achieved the goals you are working toward and can offer encouragement, insight, and advice

- the practice of saying, "Stop! ZOOM OUT," then asking yourself big-picture questions like "What really matters?" and "What do I need to see?"

- the practice of saying, "Stop! ZOOM IN," then asking yourself specific, detailed questions like "What is the best thing I can do right now?" and "How will I feel once I've cared for my own wellbeing in this way?"

- the community you've established, the supporting cast you've recruited, the relationship ecosystem you are tending to, and the circle of people who support your authentic wellbeing and prioritize their own

- the environment you've created to support the wellness rituals you've prescribed for yourself, and the boundaries you've created to protect your practice of them

That is a considerable list of wonderful resources, and I've saved the best for last: your ability to self-coach and champion your own dreams. You are the best coach for you because you know yourself best. All you must do is commit to the practice of shifting your inner narrative, stopping negative thinking in its tracks, and choosing to ask yourself empowering, constructive questions that illuminate your goals, highlight your barriers, reveal your boundaries, guide your actions, and provide accountability.

Questions are the answer to overcoming obstacles. Constructive questioning is the way to maintain the awareness that keeps you moving forward and expanding upward. These are excellent questions to ask yourself every day:

- What do I want?
- What do I know?
- What do I need to feel safe and connected?
- How will I practice?
- How did that make me feel?

The practice of asking yourself these questions will allow you to live in greater sync with your basic needs and wildest dreams. You have permission to do this, to go after what you want, and it's important that you do. When you choose this path of better wellbeing, you are applying both an instant and sustainable solution to feeling better, by abiding by your micro-manifesto and practicing the *rituals* you've learned in this book to move, nourish, rest, and connect.

I am so happy that you have arrived here, now. I truly hope this journey has provided you with more *reverence* for your life, lovingkindness for yourself, enthusiasm for your longevity, and intention for your legacy. You are the one who must choose to take good care of yourself. No one else but you can do this. And I know you can do this! I hope you feel better now, and I wish you all the best on this lifelong quest.

Acknowledgements

I AM BURSTING with thankfulness for so many people who helped me arrive at this moment. At the very top of that list is my amazing husband, partner, and best friend, Aaron. You took on so much for me to make this happen. You made great sacrifices to support me and are exceptionally generous with your thoughtful consideration, insight, and wise feedback. You always say the right thing when I am frazzled or afraid. Despite having an incredibly busy job, you took on heaps of responsibility at home so I could have most mornings to capture my peak creative time to think, research, and write. You gave me strength when I doubted myself. You have been a steadfast source of love and encouragement for the last twenty-seven years, and no words could ever convey my gratitude for having such a magnificent man in my life. Thank you from the bottom of my heart!

To my beloved daughter, Bronwyn: it is such a joy to be your mom. You have the most kind and adventurous spirit — what a gift to be your guide as you grow. Your enthusiasm, positivity, and zestiness light up every day. Please stay wild and true to your glorious, glittering self. You are a driving force in my dedication to my own well-being, as I want to be fully engaged for as much of your life as I possibly can. Thank you for the joy, meaning, and vitality you bring to my life. You are a force to behold!

Thank you to my awesome parents, Margaret and Keith, who instilled in me a love of movement, music, nature, and adventure. Mom, thank you for thousands of home-cooked meals and for your unmatched zeal for and commitment to providing me with countless extracurricular opportunities. Dad, thank you for passing on your insatiable need to explore and for giving our family so many epic adventures pretty much every weekend and summer of my childhood.

Thank you to my tremendous village of friends and family, who provide a strong foundation for me to thrive. To David, Jessica, Jeremy, Erika, Charlotte, Mariette, and Greg. To Rebecca, Jongsu, Noah, Olivia, and Conan. To Kyla and Graham. To Michele and Joel. To Lisa and Ryan. To Katherine and Chris. To Janelle and Adam. To Jill and Dave. To Erica and Michael. To Holly and Alastair. To Nichole and Jo. To Liza and Olle. To Jennifer, Cheryl, Teresa, Jodi, and Rainbow Opal Moon. I love you all so much!

Thank you to my extraordinary clients and community of alumni, especially my super alumni: Karly, Jennifer, Tiff, Erin, Tracey, and Fiona. I have learned and gained so much through my work with you. To my dream-come-true team at the Oak Bay Beach Hotel, Jennifer and Anneke, thank you for our years of creating luxury wellness retreats together. Thank you to my wise and wonderful coaches and mentors Brenda, Jessica, Bill, Carla, and Richard.

Thank you to the authors and thinkers whose work has truly inspired me, including Rick Hanson, Gabor Maté, John J. Ratey, Kelly McGonigal, Wendy Suzuki, Danielle LaPorte, Gay Hendricks, Tony Robbins, Linda Graham, Dan Buettner, Pema Chödrön, Sharon Salzberg, Phil Stutz, Amy Cuddy, Eric Goodman, Shawn Achor, Greg Wells, Michael Greger, Deborah MacNamara, Becky Kennedy, Deb Dana, Stephen Porges, Elizabeth Gilbert, Stacy Irvine, Emily Nagoski, Martha Beck, Esther Perel, Chelsey Luger, Thosh Collins, Julie Holland, Laura Vanderkam, Daniel Amen, Alex Soojung-Kim Pang, Deepak Chopra, John Sarno, James R. Doty, James Nestor, Angela Hanscom, Kimberly Ann Johnson, Arianna Huffington, Tricia Hersey, Seane Corn, Elise Loehnen, Daniel Levitin, Clarissa Pinkola Estés, Kristin Neff, Glennon Doyle, and AJ Harper.

To my brilliant Wonderwell team, Maggie, Jenn, Eva, and J, thank you for the enjoyable and illuminating experience of having you guide me through the process of creating an excellent book plan.

Thank you to my superbly talented, immensely kind, and deeply supportive Page Two team — Trena, Rony, Tass, Sarah, Adrineh, Tessa, Madelaine, and Jen — you have all made this daunting process delightfully smooth. To my wild, firecracker, heart-of-gold friend Jillian, thank you for writing the foreword to this book.

And to YOU, the reader! Thank you for giving me the opportunity to share my thoughts on wellbeing with you. I hope this book will serve you well into the future!

Notes

Introduction

7 Michael Beckwith, "Dr. Michael Beckwith on the Power of Manifestation & an Intentional Life," *The Ellen Show*, video, 8:30, October 6, 2021, https://youtu.be/ONdSvQCPjeQ.

12 *"repeated exposure to information":* John Medina, *Brain Rules: 12 Principles for Surviving and Thriving at Work, Home, and School* (Pear Press, 2014), 149, https://brainrules.net/long-term-memory.

1: Learning to Rewild

15 Clarissa Pinkola Estés, *Women Who Run with the Wolves* (Ballantine Books, 1996), 116.

19 *Integrity, the state of being whole:* Martha Beck, *The Way of Integrity: Finding the Path to Your True Self* (The Open Field, 2021), xvii.

20 *"Each of us has an inner thermostat":* Gay Hendricks, *The Big Leap: Conquer Your Hidden Fear and Take Life to the Next Level* (HarperOne, 2009), 20.

21 *"Letting yourself savour natural":* Hendricks, *The Big Leap*, 83.

23 *"Repression — dissociating emotions from awareness":* Gabor Maté, *When the Body Says No: The Cost of Hidden Stress* (Vintage Canada, 2012), 7.

2: Setting Yourself Free

31 Nelson Mandela, interview by John Battersby, *Christian Science Monitor*, February 10, 2000, https://www.csmonitor.com/2000/0210/p15s1.html.

33 *As health psychologist and author:* Kelly McGonigal, *The Upside of Stress: Why Stress Is Good for You, and How to Get Good at It* (Avery, 2015), xxi.

35 *In their book,* Burnout: Emily Nagoski and Amelia Nagoski, *Burnout: The Secret to Unlocking the Stress Cycle* (Ballantine Books, 2019), 4.

37 *In* Anchored, *licensed clinical social worker:* Deb Dana, *Anchored: How to Befriend Your Nervous System Using Polyvagal Theory* (Sounds True, 2021), 7.

3: The Life Delicious

47 Seane Corn, *Revolution of the Soul: Awaken to Love Through Raw Truth, Radical Healing, and Conscious Action* (Sounds True, 2019), 190.

48 *"What you pay attention to":* Rick Hanson, *Hardwiring Happiness: The New Brain Science of Contentment, Calm, and Confidence* (Harmony Books, 2013), 12.

51 *"Whatever we repeatedly sense":* Hanson, *Hardwiring Happiness*, 10.

61 *"Each time we switch our attention":* Daniel Levitin, interview by the author, February 1, 2015.

4: The Magic Formula

65 Gurmukh Kaur Khalsa, *Bountiful, Beautiful, Blissful* (St. Martin's Press, 2003), 17.

69 *the greatest predictors of longevity are:* Susan Pinker, "The Secret to Living Longer May Be Your Social Life," filmed April 2017, TED video, 15:52, https://www.ted.com/talks/susan_pinker_the_secret_to_living_longer_may_be_your_social_life?subtitle=en.

70 *In his TED Talk:* Shawn Achor, "The Happy Secret to Better Work," filmed May 2011 in Bloomington, IL, TED video, 12:03, https://www.ted.com/talks/shawn_achor_the_happy_secret_to_better_work.

71 *"In order to heal":* Maté, *When the Body Says No*, 24.

76 *Or you could borrow the fabulous:* Hendricks, *The Big Leap*, 156.

5: Move Your Body

83 Wendy Suzuki, *Healthy Brain, Happy Life: A Personal Program to Activate Your Brain and Do Everything Better* (Dey Street Books, 2015).

86 *recent evidence suggests that:* "What Is Sedentary Behaviour?" Sedentary Behaviour Research Network, accessed August 21, 2024, https://www.sedentarybehaviour.org/what-is-sedentary-behaviour.

87 *"We are designed to be wild":* John J. Ratey, *Go Wild: Free Your Body and Mind from the Afflictions of Civilization* (Little, Brown and Company, 2014), 4.

87 *"Movement places demands on the brain":* Ratey, *Go Wild*, 103.

89 *"In the wild, regular exercise":* Hanson, *Hardwiring Happiness*, 47.

96 *"body image has a negative impact":* "Relaxation Techniques: Breath Control Helps Quell Errant Stress Response," Harvard Health Publishing, Harvard Medical School, July 24, 2024, https://www.health.harvard.edu/mind-and-mood/relaxation-techniques-breath-control-helps-quell-errant-stress-response.

97 *"Expanding your body language":* Amy Cuddy, *Presence: Bringing Your Boldest Self to Your Biggest Challenges* (Little, Brown and Company, 2015), 216.

97 *"Power... activates a psychological":* Cuddy, *Presence,* 216.

102 *An article in the journal:* Bingqing Wang et al., "Exercise Regulates Myokines in Aging-Related Diseases through Muscle-Brain Crosstalk," *Gerontology* 70, no. 2 (February 2024): 193–209, https://doi.org/10.1159/000535339.

105 *"Physical accomplishments can change":* Kelly McGonigal, *The Joy of Movement: How Exercise Helps Us Find Happiness, Hope, Connection, and Courage* (Avery, 2021), 127.

6: Nourish Your Body

113 Deepak Chopra, *What Are You Hungry For?* (Harmony Books, 2013), 12.

115 *Hyperpalatable foods:* Tera L. Fazzino, Kaitlyn Rohde, and Debra K. Sullivan, "Hyper-Palatable Foods: Development of a Quantitative Definition and Application to the US Food System Database," *Obesity: A Research Journal* 27, no. 11 (November 2019): 1761–68, https://doi.org/10.1002/oby.22639.

119 *"Young children are restless seekers":* Deborah MacNamara, *Rest, Play, Grow: Making Sense of Preschoolers (Or Anyone Who Acts Like One)* (Aona Books, 2016), 77.

123 *The recommended dietary allowance:* "Dietary Reference Intakes Tables: Reference Values for Macronutrients," Health Canada, Government of Canada, https://www.canada.ca/en/health-canada/services/food-nutrition/healthy-eating/dietary-reference-intakes/tables/reference-values-macronutrients.html.

123 *the American College of Sports Medicine's:* Bryan Holtzman and Kathryn E. Ackerman, "Recommendations and Nutritional Considerations for Female Athletes: Health and Performance," *Sports Medicine* 51, no. S1 (September 2021): 43–57, https://doi.org/10.1007/s40279-021-01508-8.

123 *start from the current acceptable:* "Dietary Reference Intakes Tables," Health Canada.

129 *According to an article:* Michael J. Wilkinson et al., "Ten-Hour Time-Restricted Eating Reduces Weight, Blood Pressure, and Atherogenic Lipids in Patients with Metabolic Syndrome," *Cell Metabolism* 31, no. 1 (January 7, 2020): 92–104.e5, https://doi.org/10.1016/j.cmet.2019.11.004.

131 *According to the Food and Agriculture:* "Nutrition: Food Loss and Waste," Food and Agriculture Organization of the United Nations, accessed August 22, 2024, https://www.fao.org/nutrition/capacity-development/food-loss-and-waste.

131 *These losses and their associated:* United Nations Environment Programme, UNEP *Food Waste Index Report 2021*, March 2021, https://www.unep.org/resources/report/unep-food-waste-index-report-2021.

132 *Studies have linked dehydration:* Magdalena Zielińska, Edyta Łuszczki, and Katarzyna Dereń, "Dietary Nutrient Deficiencies and Risk of Depression (Review Article 2018–2023)," *Nutrients* 15, no. 11 (2023): 2433, https://doi.org/10.3390/nu15112433.

133 *organically grown fruits and vegetables:* Wisnu Adi Wicaksono et al., "The Edible Plant Microbiome: Evidence for the Occurrence of Fruit and Vegetable Bacteria in the Human Gut," *Gut Microbes* 15, no. 2 (2023): 2258565, https://doi.org/10.1080/19490976.2023.2258565.

134 *You will learn how quality sleep:* Sebastian M. Schmid et al., "A Single Night of Sleep Deprivation Increases Ghrelin Levels and Feelings of Hunger in Normal-Weight Healthy Men," *Journal of Sleep Research* 17, no. 3 (September 2008): 331–34, https://doi.org/10.1111/j.1365-2869.2008.00662.x.

7: Rest Your Body

137 Tricia Hersey, *Rest Is Resistance: A Manifesto* (Little, Brown and Spark, 2022), 8.

140 *She said that an aha moment:* An Evening with Elizabeth Gilbert in Vancouver, Queen Elizabeth Theatre, Vancouver, BC, April 14, 2023.

141 *But there's a lot more to this:* Alex Soojung-Kim Pang, *Rest: Why You Get More Done When You Work Less* (Basic Books, 2016), 74.

142 *"mind-wandering is the secret of creativity":* Pang, *Rest*, 40.

142 *"Whether they know it":* Pang, *Rest*, 47.

143 *Sleep hygiene is an important part:* World Health Organization, Health Topics, Hygiene, https://www.afro.who.int/health-topics/hygiene.

143 *A massive leap in our understanding:* Nadia Aalling Jessen et al., "The Glymphatic System – A Beginner's Guide," *Neurochemical Research* 40, no. 12 (December 2015): 2583–99, https://doi.org/10.1007/s11064-015-1581-6.

143 *In his TED Talk:* Jeffrey Iliff, "One More Reason to Get a Good Night's Sleep," filmed September 2014, TED video, 11:31, https://www.ted.com/talks/jeff_iliff_one_more_reason_to_get_a_good_night_s_sleep.

145 *And if you are curious about:* Shalini Paruthi, MD, et al., "Recommended Amount of Sleep for Pediatric Populations: A Consensus Statement of the American Academy of Sleep Medicine," *Journal of Clinical Sleep Medicine* 12, no. 6 (June 2016): 785–86, https://doi.org/10.5664/jcsm.5866.

145 *A 2024 paper in the journal:* Daniel P. Windred et al., "Sleep Regularity Is a Stronger Predictor of Mortality Risk than Sleep Duration: A Prospective Cohort Study," *Sleep* 47, no. 1 (January 2024): zsad253, https://doi.org/10.1093/sleep/zsad253.

147 *"It is hard enough for the body":* Satchin Panda, *The Circadian Code: Lose Weight, Supercharge Your Energy, and Transform Your Health from Morning to Midnight* (Rodale Books, 2018), 41.

147 *His lab studied a group:* Satchin Panda, "Circadian Code to Extend Longevity," filmed October 2017 in Venice Beach, CA, TED video, 17:03, https://www.ted.com/talks/satchin_panda_circadian_code_to_extend_longevity.

151 *When light is sensed:* Lucia Helena Souza de Toledo et al., "Modeling the Influence of Nighttime Light on Melatonin Suppression in Humans: Milestones and Perspectives," *Journal of Photochemistry and Photobiology* 16 (August 2023): 100199, https://doi.org/10.1016/j.jpap.2023.100199.

151 *Modern humans spend an average:* Nikita A. Wonga and Hamed Bahmania, "A Review of the Current State of Research on Artificial Blue Light Safety as It Applies to Digital Devices," *Heliyon* 8, no. 8 (August 2022): e10282, https://doi.org/10.1016/j.heliyon.2022.e10282.

154 *And if you're feeling groggy:* Rachel Leproult et al., "Transition from Dim to Bright Light in the Morning Induces an Immediate Elevation of Cortisol Levels," *Journal of Clinical Endocrinology & Metabolism* 86, no. 1 (January 2001): 151–57, https://doi.org/10.1210/jcem.86.1.7102.

154 *"Our liberation is deeply connected":* Hersey, *Rest Is Resistance*, 25.

8: Connect with Other Bodies

157 Audre Lorde, "Uses of the Erotic: The Erotic as Power," paper presented at the Fourth Berkshire Conference on the History of Women, Mount Holyoke College, MA, August 25, 1978.

158 *attachment is our instinct:* Gabor Maté, *The Myth of Normal: Trauma, Illness and Healing in a Toxic Culture* (Knopf Canada, 2022), 105.

160 *"Repair is one of my favourite":* Becky Kennedy, *Good Inside: A Guide to Becoming the Parent You Want to Be* (HarperCollins, 2022), 57.

160 *"Our parenting doesn't have":* Kennedy, *Good Inside*, 55.

160 *The key element of repair:* Kennedy, *Good Inside*, 58–59.

161 *"Every parent needs":* Gordon Neufeld and Gabor Maté, *Hold On to Your Kids: Why Parents Need to Matter More than Peers* (Vintage Canada, 2021), 254.

162 *"The stress of self-suppression":* Maté, *When the Body Says No*, 99.

163 *on the public health crisis:* US Department of Health and Human Services, "New Surgeon General Advisory Raises Alarm about the Devastating Impact of the Epidemic of Loneliness and Isolation in the United States," news release, May 3, 2023, https://www.hhs.gov/about/news/2023/05/03/new-surgeon-general-advisory-raises-alarm-about-devastating-impact-epidemic-loneliness-isolation-united-states.html.

163 *Positive relationships can:* Jaime Vila, "Social Support and Longevity: Meta-Analysis-Based Evidence and Psychobiological Mechanisms," *Frontiers in Psychology* 12 (2021): 717164, https://doi.org/10.3389/fpsyg.2021.717164.

164 *that stress buffer is strongest:* Vila, "Social Support and Longevity."

167 *"Love seeks closeness":* Esther Perel, *Mating in Captivity: Unlocking Erotic Intelligence* (HarperCollins, 2006), 19.

167 *"Our need for togetherness":* Perel, *Mating in Captivity*, 25.

168 *"Eroticism is a life force":* Esther Perel, "The Importance of Eroticism in Hard Times — Letters from Esther," September 15, 2021, video of online workshop streamed live, 31:08, https://www.youtube.com/live/HJ-5g3hUhNo?si=5QtVelklOTX_nYvd.

170 *morning exposure to sunlight:* Gareth Hazell, Marina Khazova, and Paul O'Mahoney, "Low-Dose Daylight Exposure Induces Nitric Oxide Release and Maintains Cell Viability In Vitro," *Scientific Reports* 13 (2023): 16306, https://doi.org/10.1038/s41598-023-43653-2.

172 *Remember that at one time:* Chelsey Luger and Thosh Collins, *The Seven Circles: Indigenous Teachings for Living Well* (HarperOne, 2022), 74.

172 *engaging with the land:* Luger and Collins, *The Seven Circles*, 94.

173 *"Every day, our relationship":* Richard Louv, *The Nature Principle: Human Restoration and the End of Nature-Deficit Disorder* (Algonquin Books, 2011), 3.

9: Zoom Out: Lovingkindness, Longevity, and Legacy

179 Maya Angelou, *Wouldn't Take Nothing for My Journey Now* (Bantam, 1994), 104.

184 *"The moment you realize":* Sharon Salzberg, *Real Happiness: The Power of Meditation* (Workman, 2011), 49.

184 *"When a thought arises":* Salzberg, *Real Happiness*, 55.

186 *The practice of meditation can:* Pema Chödrön, *How to Meditate: A Practical Guide to Making Friends with Your Mind* (Sounds True, 2013), 8.

187 *"Your wiser self is":* Linda Graham, MFT, "Cultivating the Wiser Self," accessed August 22, 204, https://lindagraham-mft.net/cultivating-the-wiser-self.

189 *"Neurostimulation is effective":* Norman Doidge, MD, *The Brain's Way of Healing* (Viking USA, 2015), 110.

190 *"The bigger idea of Blue Zones":* Dan Buettner, "I Guess I Forgot to Die: How to Defy Retirement, Boost Longevity, and Transform Your Life," August 31, 2023, in *The 1000 Hours Outside Podcast*, produced by Ginny Yurich, podcast, 51:17, https://www.1000hoursoutside.com/podcast/episode185.

10: Zoom In: Your Personal Action Plan

195 Kristin Neff, *Fierce Self-Compassion: How Women Can Harness Kindness to Speak Up, Claim Their Power, and Thrive* (Harper, 2021), 193.

201 *"Death is the most powerful":* Phil Stutz and Barry Michels, *The Tools: 5 Tools to Help You Find Courage, Creativity, and Willpower—and Inspire You to Live Life in Forward Motion* (Random House, 2013), 200.

201 *"Your future is in jeopardy"*: Stutz and Michels, *The Tools*, 198.

Conclusion

205 Elizabeth Gilbert, *Big Magic: Creative Living Beyond Fear* (Riverhead Books, 2015), 101.

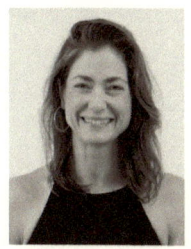

About the Author

CATHERINE ROSCOE BARR is a neuroscience-based wellness coach and founder of The Life Delicious, an evidence-based curriculum of sustainable practices grounded in pleasure and simplicity to liberate ourselves and others from suffering. Roscoe Barr offers women's coaching circles, co-ed retreats, corporate workshops, and keynote speeches; is a certified personal trainer, fitness instructor, and coach practitioner; and writes about fitness, food, and travel for numerous print and online publications. Before settling on the West Coast, she lived in Sydney, Toronto, Oregon, Montana, and practically everywhere in Alberta. She currently lives in Vancouver with her fabulous husband, delightful daughter, and adorable dog.

READY TO HELP YOUR TEAM
FEEL BETTER NOW?

HERE ARE FOUR WAYS I CAN SHARE THIS WELLNESS REVOLUTION WITH YOU:

- **Conference keynote:** I can uplift, invigorate, and engage your attendees with practical and inspiring takeaways.

- **Wellness retreat:** I can whisk you and your team away to a luxury property where you'll be nourished and pampered as you engage in an immersive learning experience.

- **Corporate workshop series (online or in person):** I can empower your organization with evidence-based practices for physical and psychological wellbeing through an extended learning journey.

- **Bulk orders:** For bulk orders of *Feel Better Now*, please contact orders@pagetwo.com.

Let's do this! Contact me through my website at thelifedelicious.ca to get started.

www.ingramcontent.com/pod-product-compliance
Lightning Source LLC
Chambersburg PA
CBHW060559080526
44585CB00013B/617